RHETORICS OF REFUSAL

RHETORICS OF REFUSAL

MEDICAL DISSENT AND THE US-SOMALI DIASPORA

Kari Campeau

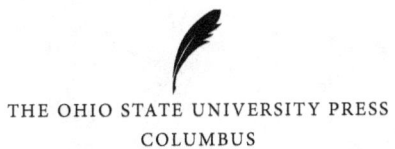

THE OHIO STATE UNIVERSITY PRESS
COLUMBUS

Copyright © 2025 by The Ohio State University.
All rights reserved.

Library of Congress Cataloging-in-Publication data available online at https://catalog.loc.gov
LCCN: 2025011033
Identifiers: ISBN 9780814215883 (hardback); ISBN 9780814259467 (paperback); ISBN 9780814284155 (ebook)

Cover design by Laurence J. Nozik
Text composition by Stuart Rodriguez
Type set in Minion Pro

CONTENTS

Acknowledgments	vii
INTRODUCTION	1
Explaining (Away) "No": Studying Dissent in Medicine and the Humanities	6
Rhetorical Refusal	24
The Study, Site, and Methods	31
About Autism	36
Review of the Chapters	38
CHAPTER 1 Welcome to Health Class: Community Sickness as Rhetorical Refusal's Fertile Ground	41
A New Health Literacy Course: Preparation, Delivery, Evaluation, and Tensions	43
Five Discourses of Autism as Community Sickness	54
Rhetorical Refusal through Wrong Discourses	67
Community Sickness as Rhetorical Refusal's Fertile Ground	70
Conclusion	71

CHAPTER 2 Outbreak: Vaccine Dissent as Embodied Rhetorical Refusal	72
Historical Vaccine Frames and the Rise of the Racialized Wrong-Belief Frame	75
Somali Stories of the Minnesota Measles Outbreak	88
Tracing Rhetorical Refusal's Arc through Vaccine Dissent	100
Conclusion	108
CHAPTER 3 Writing to the State: Mistakes and Silences as Rhetorical Refusal	110
Public Assistance: Diaspora Visions and Resettled Realities	112
The Paperwork: Outreach Materials, the Grant Application, and a Consumer-Directed Model of Care	116
Rhetorical Refusals through Mistakes, Silences, and Departures	119
Rhetorical Refusal in Institutional Documentation	141
Conclusion	145
CHAPTER 4 The Persuasive Microbiome: Rhetorical Refusal through Care	147
Who Is the Microbiome For? Popular and Scientific Discourses of the Microbiome	148
Nasra's Story	158
Five Topoi across Microbiome Stories	165
Following Refusal's Arc: The Microbiome's Health Futures	179
A Five-Topoi Framework for Listening to Medical Dissent as Rhetorical Refusal	182
Conclusion	184
CONCLUSION	186
References	193
Index	209

ACKNOWLEDGMENTS

Thank you to everyone who participated in the research for this book. To the parents who participated in this study, thank you for sharing parts of your lives, homes, and stories with me. To those at Midnimo, thank you for the friendship and for the opportunity to work together. Thank you for teaching me a new orientation to research, one grounded in accountability and community. It was an honor to work alongside you all. Thank you to the public health professionals, social service professionals, community health workers, healthcare providers, public school liaisons, and activists who shared your knowledge, experiences, and glimpses of your working worlds with me. Thank you, too, for your tireless work in the service of community health and healthcare access. I hope this book can support your work.

Thank you to my mentors, colleagues, and students at the Department of Writing Studies at the University of Minnesota. Thank you, Mary Lay Schuster; your scholarship was a guiding light for me long before I ever imagined I would have the opportunity to work with you. Your work and mentorship keep me focused on the relationship between rhetoric and advocacy and on what research can do in the world. Thank you, Lee-Ann Kastman Breuch, Karen-Sue Taussig, and Molly Kessler; your feedback and insights on this project allowed me to make connections and arguments that otherwise I would not have made and helped me push my analyses to new places. Thank you to my colleagues, especially Alexander Champoux-Crowley, Niki Cuilla, Evelyn

Dsouza, Ryan Eichberger, McKinley Green, and Juliette Lapeyrouse-Cherry, for your intellectual companionship, for opportunities to read your scholarship, and for feedback on this project in its early stages. A huge thank-you to my students for bringing fresh perspectives and helping me see rhetoric and medical scholarship in new ways.

I want to thank the University of Minnesota, Social Science Research Council, and Bush Headwaters Foundation for the financial support. Community-based fieldwork takes time and involves unpredictable timelines and outcomes, and I would not have been able to do this partnered research without these funding sources.

I have had opportunities to present and receive meaningful feedback on parts of this project at conferences, including those hosted by the Association for the Rhetoric of Science, Technology, and Medicine; Association of Teachers of Technical Writing; and the American Society of Bioethics and Humanities. I have published articles related to this research in two journals, the editors and reviewers of which helped guide this book's argument. At *Rhetoric of Health and Medicine,* thank you to Lisa Melonçon, Cathryn Molloy, and the anonymous reviewers, whose questions and feedback led me to think about nonvaccination as a form of rhetorical participation. At *Journal of Technical Writing and Communication,* thank you to themed issue editor Kirk St. Amant for your guidance on my article on person-centered care.

Thank you to those who made the publication of this book possible. Thank you to Tara Cyphers, my editor at The Ohio State University Press, for your investment in this book's possibilities and your insights as I revised. Thank you to the two anonymous readers, whose generous feedback was instrumental to my revisions; your feedback helped me clarify rhetorical refusal as a concept, push my argument to make bolder claims about medical dissent, and reorganize the manuscript to make a stronger argument. I aspire to be such a careful, generative, and supportive reader for fellow scholars' work.

I first began thinking about rhetoric, vaccination, and the nuances of medical dissent in class with Bernice Hausman at Virginia Tech University. Little did I know that this class would shape my scholarly identity and research path for years to come. Bernice Hausman, thank you for your mentorship and your scholarship. Thank you for welcoming me into the Vaccination Research Group, where I learned about the possibilities of research in the medical humanities as well as how to do humanistic research. I returned to your books and articles and to my notes from your lectures and the VRG many times while researching, writing, and revising this book; I am so grateful that your work and perspectives are foundational to my research and writing. I was also so fortunate to get to work with Heidi Lawrence at the Vaccine

Research Group and beyond. Heidi Lawrence, thank you for your mentorship, friendship, and scholarship. You might not remember this, but thank you for welcoming me to present work with you at ARSTM when I was a new graduate student. I continue to learn so much from your work.

Thank you to my colleagues and students at University of Colorado, Denver. Thank you to the English Department for being a great place to work, teach, and write. Thank you to Jennifer Reich for your work on vaccination and for taking the time to listen to my ideas, provide feedback, and for encouraging me to see this project through. Thank you to John Tinnell for your advice on walks around Sloans and for helping me navigate this project. Thank you to my students for trusting me with your insights, intellectual work, and your personal and professional goals.

Thank you to the childcare professionals and teachers who took care of my children and helped them grow and learn. Without you, I never would not have had the time and focus to finish this book.

Thank you to my family. Puttermans, thanks to you all, I have never doubted that I have people who believe in me and who will be there for me, no matter what. Mum, I love sharing time, lunches, and conversation with you; you always keep me centered. Dad, I am grateful for our relationship and how it has grown. To Sara, my sister, thank you for being my best friend and for being by my side, no matter what. Nathan, thank you for everything; you live out what it means to be a partner, through thick and thin. Addie and Jack, I love you both, forever and ever.

INTRODUCTION

"Autism," Waris, a Somali mother who came to Minneapolis, Minnesota, as a refugee twelve years ago, explained to me, "is our community's sickness."

"Somalia," Kadra said, "is a country of poets, and here my child can't speak."

"I see my son as a blessing," Fartun explained, "and I need to care for him. Sometimes he runs away because he's in his own head. It's just, I can't describe it, but he goes somewhere else, his brain goes into its own world, and he can get lost. Every time he comes back, I could yell at him, but I just hug him. I rub his back."

"It's everything," Farax said. "Vaccines, climate, where we live, what we eat. Everything is making our children sick."

"My husband and my brother, they said, he's just different than the others, he's fine," Sofia explained about her young son. "He'll talk when he's ready. If you take him in, they'll measure everything, and they'll find something wrong with him."

"I want resources for my daughter," Asma told me.

"I feel like a cat," Nasra told me. "At parent-teacher conferences, I feel like a cat. I want to lunge across the table, and I want to scream, don't you see he's different?

Now, at conferences, I ask everyone to pray with me. I say, let's do this. All of us, let's close our eyes. I say all of us are gathered to help Zeki do his best."

"I want to keep track of everything," Kowsar explained as she set a white binder in front of me. Inside, she had hole-punched and organized every written communication about her son's autism. "I do it for myself because there is so much, but for other mothers, too. Everything takes so long. Today, I was on hold for over two hours. Two hours and 31 minutes, and then it just hung up on me. I'm going to write a book, eventually."

"He must go to college first," Anab said. "I have this vision: his math scores are very high, and if we can get his reading scores higher, he could go to college, study math. I cry when I think of my son getting a scholarship and going to college."

"I would like to go to school, too," Dehka said, "and I would study research."

On Monday, April 10, 2017, the Minnesota Department of Health (MDH) received a report that a 25-month-old child had been hospitalized with a rash and fever. This incident would be recognized as the first measles case of what would become Minnesota's largest outbreak since 1990. The outbreak resulted in 75 measles cases, most of which (68 cases, 91%) occurred in Somali children who had not received the recommended two dosages of the measles-mumps-rubella (MMR) vaccine.[1] Ten years prior to the outbreak, however, Somali children[2] made up one of the most reliably vaccinated populations in the state; MMR vaccination coverage rates for children of Somali descent regularly exceeded 95 percent. By 2011, the MMR vaccination rate among Minnesota's Somali children had dropped to 54 percent and, by 2014, to 46 percent. Meanwhile, the rate among non-Somali Minnesotan two-year-old children was 88 percent. By 2016, the rate of MMR vaccination in Somali children statewide had fallen to 42 percent (Banerjee et al., 2020). In April 2017, Minnesota was embroiled in a measles outbreak.

---

1. The median age for all cases was two years (range: three months to 57 years). Sixty-one (81%) cases were of Somali descent; one (1%) was Black and of non-Somali descent; two (3%) were white, Hispanic; and 11 (15%) were white, non-Hispanic. The measles cases were transmitted in childcare (n = 32), household (n = 26), school (n = 4), healthcare (n = 2), community (n = 10), and unknown (n = 1) settings (MDH, 2017).

2. The collapse of the Somali state in 1991 led to mass migration, and that migration continues today. Many Somalis have come to Minnesota as refugees of civil warfare, famine, and state collapse in Somalia. Somali refugees came to the US from long-term refugee camps in Northeastern Africa; now, Minneapolis is home to the largest Somali population in the US.

Public health accounts and news media coverage largely attributed the decline in Somali vaccination rates to predatory moves by antivaccination groups who capitalized on Somali concerns about autism in the Western diaspora. Indeed, 2008, the year that Somali vaccination rates began to drop, was also when Somali parents began speaking out about what they suspected were unexplained clusters of autism among Somali youth living in the Western diaspora. In Minnesota, Somali parent advocacy groups pressed MDH for answers as to why so many of their children were being diagnosed at school with autism (Hewitt et al., 2016). Their efforts compelled several research studies (Hewitt et al., 2013; Hewitt et al., 2016) *and* caught the attention of antivaccination advocates.

Beginning in 2008, antivaccination leaders visited Minneapolis multiple times and held events at Somali gathering spots (Sun, 2017; Sohn, 2017). When the measles outbreak took hold in Minnesota, these antivaccination visits persisted and took center stage in media coverage of the outbreak. CNN introduced the outbreak to its global readership, "Antivaccine groups blamed in Minnesota measles outbreak" (Howard, 2017). The *Washington Post* reported: "Antivaccine activists spark a state's worst measles outbreak in decades" (Sun, 2017). *Vox* told the story of "why Minnesota lost a battle against antivaccine campaigners" (Belluz, 2017). Across local and national headlines, a narrative took shape: antivaccination predators were exploiting a vulnerable population. Public health accounts of the outbreak advanced a similar story. Minnesota's state health commissioner, Ed Ehlinger, blamed the outbreak on the targeted dissemination of disinformation in his public statement, which began, "Unfortunately, the Minnesota Somali community has been targeted with misinformation about vaccine risks" (Dyer, 2017). State epidemiologist Kristen Ehresmann described the turning point in Somali vaccine behavior as wrought by the arrival of antivaccine activists: "What's very striking is that when you look at before and after that point in time, you can see the impact that the antivaccine groups have had on the community. I'll be honest. It makes me very angry" (Branswell, 2017). "It's remarkable," Siman Nuurali, a Somali American clinician at Children's Hospitals and Clinics of Minnesota, told the *Washington Post* in reference to antivaccination leaders, "to come in and talk to a population that's vulnerable and marginalized and who doesn't necessarily have the capacity for advocacy for themselves, and to take advantage of that. It's abhorrent" (as qtd. in Sun, 2017).

The published record of the 2017 measles outbreak tells a consistent story. Antivaccination charlatans invaded a community and took advantage of its vulnerable members. They exploited fear and sowed uncertainty. They spread disinformation. They incited an infectious disease outbreak. This story makes logical certain solutions. Namely, disinformation must be combated. Accordingly, public health leaders and organizations committed to building stronger relationships with Somali organizations, conducting more outreach to Somali Minnesotans, and communicating accurate and culturally specific information to their Somali community members. By many metrics, these public health interventions worked. The outbreak was contained. There were no fatalities. In the years following the outbreak, vaccination rates of Somali American children climbed (Richert, 2018).

But this is a partial story. Also during the 2017 Minnesota measles outbreak, I was working as a researcher with a Somali women's health center in Minneapolis called Midnimo (a pseudonym[3]), and I couldn't shake the knowledge that the stories I heard from Somali parents at the health center were very different from the stories populating the public discourse. At the health center, there was little discussion of antivaccination groups. Although I knew many parents who declined, selectively declined, or delayed vaccinations, rarely were parents confident that the MMR vaccine would cause autism. Rarely could parents' concerns be traced back to an antivaccine talking point. The stories I heard were layered, ambivalent, and shifting. They were stories told by frustrated, activist, and determined parents making and remaking complex health decisions. In interviews, Somali American parents weighed whether they should trust the recommendations produced by an expensive healthcare system that seemed impervious to their needs. Somali American parents explained that much remained unknown about the somatic residues of displacement, forced migration, and ongoing precarity. Parents expressed concerns that their children had received multiple rounds of the same vaccine at refugee camps and upon resettlement. Was there clinical research that spoke to refugee-specific embodied experiences, including but not limited to vaccination? Parents spoke to the need to protect their children and to the feeling that they had only inaccessible medical tools to do so and scraps of information. The stories I heard were, on the surface, about vaccination and autism. But they were also stories of mothers managing somatic differences in an unstable world. Stories of parents entering and being repelled or surveilled by an unfamiliar medical system. Stories about promises and disappointments. Stories abuzz with rumored theories and experiential hunches; stories interspersed with technical medical diagnoses preserved in plastic sleeves and stored on closet shelves. They were stories about children becoming themselves and engaging with their worlds, stories about fierce sibling friendships, about children's bright minds, and about family memories. They were stories

---

3. All names of participants and specific locations are pseudonyms.

brimming with questions—how to make sense of disability and medicine and all the technical language that goes into making these categories actionable? They were stories of families mediating between modes of health knowledge to make sense of somatic changes. Stories laced the lurking knowledge of how loss and trauma burrow into and mark bodies through generations. They were stories about hope. Hope for resources, for health, for education, for change, for listeners, for home.

These stories could not be squared with the exploited, silent parents depicted in news coverage and in public health assessments of the measles outbreak. As well, these complex concerns were not assuaged by MDH's targeted vaccine-messaging campaigns. Somali American parents' concerns persisted, even as some parents consented to vaccines. One Somali American mother, participating in an interview with me, related her memory of getting her son vaccinated with the MMR vaccine right on schedule, on his first birthday: "My husband and I," she recalled, "we watched all day holding our breath. We stared at him as he slept. We didn't speak. I remember every second. We were waiting, is he going to change? Will it happen to him? We were waiting for him to stop speaking, to freeze up. You know, how others say it happens: the light disappears from his eyes. We were waiting to lose him" (3/23/2018).

I asked how she felt now, months later, and her son showed no negative effects. She said, "Lucky."

This was not trust. This was, as another Somali American mother described, "jumping from one fire to another" (3/2/2018). In talking with Somali American parents as well as public health professionals, community health workers, healthcare providers, and Somali activists, I came to understand that targeted antivaccine disinformation campaigns were only one slice of the story. As humanist Bernice L. Hausman (2019) has argued, antivaccination beliefs rarely catch on through exposure. There must be "fertile ground for vaccine skepticism to flourish" (p. 18). Or, as Anab Gulaid, a public health researcher at the University of Minnesota's Institute on Community Integration, explained about Somali vaccine hesitancy, "There is a context; this didn't just come out of nowhere" (as qtd. in Sohn, 2017).

This project began as a way to listen to the "fertile ground" or "context" that fostered Somali American parents' vaccine refusals. The project grew to include related medical dissent, and the chapters that follow engage stories from four different sites of dissent: a community-run health literacy class, the 2017 measles outbreak, a new state program to provide Somali American families with autism-related resources, and microbiome-informed naturopathic care. In these four sites, Somali American parents refused mainstream medical evidence, guidance, and resources. As well, in each of these sites,

Somali American parents' uncertainties, withdrawals, and refusals were read, in the public discourse, as remediable consequences of scientific literacy deficits and disinformation or misinformation. But not all acts of medical dissent are symptoms of a lack of scientific knowledge. In this book, I develop the concept of rhetorical refusal to recognize dissent as rhetorical, agentive, meaningful, and communicative. Sometimes refusal is an affiliative act, one that turns inward as a form of protection for community, family, or self. Other times, refusal is participatory, a strategy that marginalized rhetors use to craft public-facing, activist arguments. Rhetorical refusal is an especially necessary communicative move in places where power is uneven and oppressive; where people from marginalized groups are denied credibility, authority, and rhetorical platform; and where speaking and publicity can bring harm, surveillance, and risk. In these power-corroded discursive spaces, rhetoric—communication, argument, meaning-making, disruptions of meaning-making—is constrained but still happens, just through modes not widely recognized as rhetorical: a declined vaccine, a missed doctor's appointment, an incomplete medical intake form, a complete but unsubmitted proposal for state aid. These and other acts, if recognized as rhetorical, have much to say, argue, and envision.

Indeed, rhetorical refusals happen at a level that is rarely seen as rhetorical or agentive; as such, refusals are often misread as fixable signs of deficit. But rhetorical refusals respond to and illuminate how scientific knowledge descends into people's everyday lives, in ways that benefit some people and ask others to take on disproportionate risks. This book argues for the importance of following rhetorical refusals as participatory and protective strategies that can hold institutions accountable, advocate for change, and carve out ways to practice care differently. Before returning to the concept of rhetorical refusal, I map dominant approaches to medical dissent in medicine, public health, and the humanities and social sciences. These following sections consider the logics and histories that have informed dominant approaches to medical dissent.

Explaining (Away) "No": Studying Dissent in Medicine and the Humanities

How to understand medical dissent? How to respond to arguments and beliefs about health, illness, and the body that are not grounded in scientific evidence? Why do some people turn down healthcare? These questions inform this book's advancement of rhetorical refusal as a concept to listen to and by which to learn from medical dissent. But first it is important to engage with other foundational frames that have shaped public understandings of, institutional and interpersonal responses to, and research concerning medical dissent. In medicine, the terms *compliance, nonadherence, nonconcordance,* and *hesitancy* have been used to name dissent; in response, literacy, culture, and trust are mainstream frames used to explain and solve dissent. Outside of medicine, *resistance, refusal,* and *suspicion* have been taken up in the social sciences and humanities to theorize medical dissent. These three terms address instances of saying no, not only as negations but also as creative openings conducive to learning from dissident voices and nonstandard epistemologies. The following subsections engage with these sets of terms and how they frame dissent.

Medical Approaches to Naming "No": Compliance, Concordance, Adherence, and Hesitancy

Compliance

Cohering in the United States in the 1950s, the medical discourse of compliance took hold as a primary way to understand patients' deviations from medical instructions. Medical humanist Jeremy A. Greene's historical investigation of the term's emergence shows that noncompliance subsumed a more situation-specific gamut of terms used to describe "difficult" patients. For example, tuberculosis patients in the 1900s who did not abide by hygienic protocols were "careless," "irresponsible," and "deviant." Psychiatric patients who questioned new-to-the-scene psychopharmaceutical agents were "difficult." Pregnant women who did not keep up with their prescribed iron supplements were "non cooperative" (2004, p. 331). Importantly, such labels were often elided with other markers of difference, as patients who were poor or immigrants were judged as morally deviant or medically uneducated, while patients who were white, male, and affluent were given more leeway to exercise their opinions in medical encounters (p. 332). These various terms, while morally laden and used to further stigmatize marginalized populations, were also used situationally, to study instances of deviation in their own contexts, as enacted by specific people in response to specific disease entities and experiences.

That specificity faded under the new clinical designation of noncompliance. The rewriting of these circumstantial instances of individual refusal into a generalized category of noncompliance blurred specificity and sidelined considerations of context (Martins, 2006). Noncompliant patients were those who did not follow a physician's orders (M. S. Davis, 1968; Trostle, 1997). They were categorically in the wrong. By the 1970s, discussions of compliance had migrated from specialty journals to general medical journals, wherein noncompliance was handled as a "unique pathological entity" that cut across patient populations and disease experiences (Greene, 2004, p. 332). In Greene's summation: "This therapeutic infidelity [noncompliance] was abstracted away from the life-experience of individual patients and placed on the table as a research subject, dressed and prepared for dissection" (2004, p. 329).

Rhetorician Catherine Gouge (2018) has also argued that the automatic valuation and assumption of patient compliance necessitates abstracting patients' healthcare actions from their contexts, from the sociohistorical, political, and discursive-material contexts in which people apply medical knowledge and practice care. Gouge aligns the "privileged position of compliance" to that of "whiteness, the able body, and masculinity" and argues that the assumption of compliance is an "exclusionary fantasy" that not only oversimplifies the contexts of patients but ignores the reality that noncompliance itself is normal—how often does a person follow all medical directions and recommendations as prescribed? Still, compliance "is presumed to be the responsible, ethical, and capable condition of ideal patients," such that compliance remains "the norm against which noncompliance can be defined as deviant or immoral, something to be measured and corrected" (pp. 123, 125). With little rhetorical space to address the gradations and contexts of noncompliance, noncompliant patients blur into a standardized group that requires management and correction.

How did compliance come to occupy this position as an "unmarked norm" in biomedicine, an obvious ethical and right action (Gouge, 2018, p. 123)? Greene's work offers several reasons for the dominance of *noncompliance* as a catch-all term for dissent. First, new pharmaceutical technologies of surveillance (counting pills, laboratory tests) allowed doctors to monitor, with little to no direct interactions with patients, the extent to which patients were complying or not with their prescriptions. Second, a spike in noncompliance concern was also a response to increasing numbers of malpractice suits against providers. Just as new technologies allowed physicians to track patients' compliance, so too did new technologies bring new ways to blame physicians for not doing enough to help a patient. In an increasingly litigious healthcare space, noncompliance proved a useful legal tactic to protect physicians and place blame on patients gone rogue. Thirdly, patient noncompliance was used to combat mounting critiques of medicine, such as those of the patient autonomy and women's health movements in the 1960s and 1970s (Greene, 2004).

Gouge's work (2018) has further shown how the expectations of compliance have endured and, if anything, expanded as diseases and medicine have changed; Gouge uses the term "Compliance 1.0" to refer to the expectation that sick patients should follow medical guidance in their assumed quest to regain health (pp. 118–119). However, as the incidence of chronic illness has risen alongside the advancements of medicine and preventative care, the nature of patienthood has shifted such that the typical patient is no longer the sick patient but the at-risk patient, and being a good patient involves not just following treatment orders when one is sick but surveilling, in health and sickness, one's body along medical metrics, noticing and acting on risk, and optimizing health. Enter "Compliance 2.0," which requires that "we consent to our construction as overdetermined, medicalized subjects—even before we are ill" and in which "anyone who fails to be proactive, anyone who fails to follow the 'best practices' to prevent the onset of illness, is implicated" (p. 120). Noncompliance, then, is grounded in the assumption of a standard body and the existence of known, disease-specific pathways to health; at the same name, noncompliance, as a concept, has proven flexible, for it has endured as models of medicine, health, and patienthood have evolved. As models of health and medicine have changed, and as the practices involved in compliance have changed, compliance itself remains an "unquestioned ideal," one that glides along "largely unexamined in Western biomedicine as the 'unmarked normal'" (Gouge, 2018, p. 123). In turn, noncompliance has consistently labeled those who refuse medicine as wrong and has consistently refocused structural critiques into concerns for individual compliance.

Concordance and Adherence

Noncompliance, as a term, was useful to shore up medicine's authority, but, for this reason as well, it fell out of vogue. As medicine aimed for more patient-centered, collaborative, and culturally informed practices, *compliance* gave way to less paternalistic terms, including *concordance, adherence,* and *hesitancy*. Because *noncompliance* functioned to consolidate medical authority, the term also garnered criticism for its paternalism and underlying assumptions of patient passivity and ignorance (Conrad, 1985; Trostle, 1988; Aronson, 2007). For these reasons, *compliance* was joined in the mid-1990s by *concordance* and *adherence,* terms that were positioned as less authoritarian and more progressive (Mullen, 1997; Trostle, 1997; Segal, 2007). These terms were commonly used to foreground the role of patients as active participants in their healthcare (Segal, 2007).

Health policy scholar Daniel Skinner and medical sociologist Berkeley Franz (2018) have argued that these new terms, even as they sought to attune researchers and clinicians to the reasons patients might not comply, were limited in that they remained centered on the physician-patient relationship and in that they assumed that patient compliance was the end goal, even if it could be worthwhile to consider *why* some patients didn't comply. So long as the private patient-provider relationship was at the core of noncompliance studies, researchers would look toward interventions at the individual level. The terms *nonconcordance* and *nonadherence* were consistent with the model of noncompliance in that they kept responsibility for medicine uptake and efficiency on patients and their individual beliefs and decisions, rather than on medical systems (Charles, 2022, p. 6). Skinner and Franz (2018) have argued that concordance and adherence functioned as mere "rhetorical repackagings" that hid and thereby neutralized the interests of the compliance model (p. 242); these new terms "served at the same time to validate physician dominance within medicine and reassert the medical encounter as fundamentally individualistic" (p. 242).

Hesitancy

Hesitancy also arose as a progressive alternative for *noncompliance*. *Hesitancy* has been used mostly in relation to nonvaccination. *Vaccine hesitancy* has served as a more agreeable alternative to colloquial and pejorative terms such as *antivaccination* or *antivaxxer*. The term was popularized in 2019, when the World Health Organization (WHO) identified vaccine hesitancy as one of ten top global health threats. WHO defined vaccine hesitancy as "the reluctance or refusal to vaccinate despite the availability of vaccines" (2019). Vaccine hesitancy encompasses decisions to refuse all vaccines, refuse some vaccines, delay all or some vaccines, or accept vaccines with trepidation. The term therefore centers the complexity of vaccine doubts. From this premise, WHO advanced a "3Cs" conceptual model for understanding vaccine hesitancy; the "3Cs" model identifies the following three sources of vaccination behavior: (1) confidence, or trust in the safety and effectiveness of vaccines and the systems that study and deliver vaccines; (2) complacency, or assessments of whether a particular vaccine against a particular disease is necessary; and (3) convenience, or the extent to which vaccines and information are accessible and affordable (2019, pp. 10–11). The 3Cs model has contributed to a shift in public health approaches to vaccine hesitancy as informed not only by knowledge deficits but also by a complex interplay of economic, political, and sociocultural factors, including history, politics, religion, mode of delivery, experiences with the pharmaceutical industry, and experiences with health systems (Larson, 2020). Still, historian Nicole Charles (2022) has pointed out that *hesitancy* is limited in that the term lives squarely within a biomedical framework, one that assumes that vaccine confidence is always the right stance, even if people deviate from that stance for complex reasons. Charles has argued that hesitancy is not a far departure from deficit-based noncompliance approaches because hesitancy situates any departure from medical recommendations as informed by a remediable lack (pp. 27–29). The vaccine-hesitant make their decisions because of a *lack of confidence* in science. They put off vaccinating because of a *lack of urgency* about a particular vaccine or disease risk. They fail to vaccinate because of a *lack of access* to good information. And these lacks call for prompt correction.

Together, these terms—*compliance, concordance, adherence, hesitancy*—have guided medical and public health approaches to dissent and uncertainty. They tell a story of a mid-century contraction of noncompliant acts from idiosyncratic, situation-specific, and bias-inflected into the general category of noncompliance. As medicine aimed for more patient-centered, collaborative, and culturally informed practices, noncompliance gave way to less judgmental but still homogenizing terms, including *adherence, concordance,* and *hesitancy.* These terms were not as abrasive as compliance, but they still worked within a biomedical worldview and from the premise that individual compliance was the goal. Too, these terms and their worldviews make legible certain solutions. In the next section, I explain how these ways of understanding a patient's "no" orient investment in three types of solutions, all three of which focus on individual beliefs and decision-making.

Medical Approaches to Explaining "No": Literacy, Culture, and Trust

Compliance, concordance, adherence, and *hesitancy* name and define what it means for a patient to waver or dissent in a medical encounter. *Compliance, adherence, concordance,* and *hesitancy* all frame patient dissent or divergence as a problem to be solved. The assumption across these frames is that following medical directions is "the right path, the ethical imperative, evidence of effective coping" (Gouge, 2018, p. 123). In these frames, too, noncompliance is cast as deviant, as a barrier to care, and so "part of the role of health-care professionals is to manage and sometimes mediate individuals' self-destructive tendencies so that they can be saved from themselves" (Gouge, 2018, pp. 114–115). The next set of frames—literacy, culture, and trust—are ones used to explain noncompliance and, accordingly, to prescribe paths to managing and, ideally, eliminating noncompliance.

This set of frames—literacy, culture, and trust—reckon with why people say no to medicine. Each explains why patients dissent and identifies logical pathways to compliance and improved health outcomes. These frames seek to identify root causes of dissent that can then be targeted and solved.

Literacy

Health literacy refers to a person's ability to understand and use available health information and medical services for maximum benefit. Health literacy gained traction in Western medical spaces in the early 1970s and was defined primarily as an individual capacity or deficiency (Gele et al., 2016). Increasingly, health literacy has been addressed, too, on the systemic level, as a capacity that should be cultivated across patients, providers, and organizations, all of which have a role to play in building spaces where people can make informed decisions about their health. To this effect, the Office of Disease Prevention and Health Promotion (within the US Department of Health and Human Services), in their "Healthy People 2030" report, identified two definitions of health literacy (definitions that have been adopted by the National Institutes of Health [NIH], Centers for Disease Control [CDC], and Agency for Healthcare Research and Quality [AHRQ]): personal health literacy, "the degree to which individuals have the ability to find, understand, and use information and services to inform health-related decisions and actions for themselves and others," and organizational health literacy, "the degree to which organizations equitably enable individuals to find, understand, and use information and services to inform health-related decisions and actions for themselves and others" (Office of Disease Prevention and Health Promotion, 2020; NIH, 2021). WHO has also adopted an expansive definition of health literacy, as composed of the environmental, political, and social factors that determine health, as well as personal skills and competencies that individuals develop over their lifetimes to find, comprehend, evaluate, and use health information to make healthful decisions (Kickbusch et al., 2013). These definitions suggest that health literacy is widely framed as an individual capacity, but one that is shaped by broader contexts and cultivated within organizations and institutions.

It follows that health literacy is widely identified as a contributor to health disparities. Deficits in health literacy correlate with negative health outcomes (Meyer, Yoon, and Kaufmann, 2013), and there is significant overlap in the demographic characteristics of those who have low health literacy and those who are overrepresented in health disparities and bear the most burden of chronic illnesses and disease. In the US, factors such as lower income or education, lack of health insurance coverage, older age, and lower levels of English language proficiency have been found to be associated with lower levels of health literacy (AHRQ, 2008; Hickey et al., 2008; NIH, 2021; Keene Woods et al., 2023). Accordingly, low health literacy rates have been the focus of national initiatives, as well as state and local ones. In Minnesota, the Minnesota Health Literacy Partnership partners with major healthcare providers to practice "consumer-focused health literacy" (Minnesota Health Literacy Partnership, 2016), and the Mayo Clinic hosts the Somali Health Literacy Project, which holds monthly educational trainings for Somali residents (American Hospital Association, 2016). Researchers have tested literacy interventions such as video delivery of health information (Sunni et al., 2023), health-related comics (Garrison-Joyner and Caravella, 2020), community-based health literacy classes (Mulcahy et al., 2019), and story-based health-education interventions (Njeru et al., 2015). Many of these health literacy interventions have resulted in more accessible healthcare and better health outcomes.

At the same time, health literacy, as a frame, can risk rewriting health inequities into a problem of literacy. The literacy frame explains that people reject or equivocate about medicine because they don't know enough about medicine, and so the solution is clear: teach people about science so that they can understand, appreciate, and comply with medical guidance. The health literacy frame focuses on information, the content of science and medicine, and less often considers science as a human, social, economic, and political activity. Charles's study of HPV vaccine refusal in Barbados (2022) is an instructive example of the limits of health literacy as an explanatory framework. Global public health agencies blamed Afro-Barbadians' low uptake of the HPV vaccine on their low health literacy and resultant susceptibility to myths and fear-mongering about unsubstantiated dangers of the HPV vaccine, but Charles shows that negative attitudes about the new vaccine were more informed by a keen knowledge of past violations brought by global biotechnologies and their proponents, including "histories of biomedical surveillance, pharmaceutical experimentation, and profit of and on Black women's bodies" (p. 62). Afro-Barbadian parents did not misunderstand science. Parents' deep, lived understandings of public health as a "colonial biopolitical project" taught them to distrust public health approaches to risk and intervention. Afro-Barbadian parents' contexts of health decision-making and risk deliberation could not be addressed in a health literacy framework because the health literacy framework often atomizes historical contexts and wrongs into problems of individual comprehension such that the legible response is more information, more education. Further depicting how the health literacy framework can be a silencing one, technical communication scholar Isidore K. Dorpenyo (2022) has argued that people with alternative views about biotechnologies are often labeled as "illiterate" to delegitimize "unneeded or unwanted knowledge" (p. 305). Dorpenyo expands on the connotations of illiteracy: "In a postcolonial context, [illiteracy] could mean the referent has not acquired the proper form of education, that is, the western form of education. That individual, thus, is considered backward, primitive, and culturally stagnant" (p. 305). Dorpenyo warns that the health literacy framework is useful to label all non-Western, nonscientific health beliefs as wrong and to diminish the knowledge, perspectives, and voices of those who speak outside of Western and scientific models of health and care. The health literacy frame can easily be applied too widely and can rewrite all nonscientific beliefs and actions as fixable errors, informed only by wrong information and never by histories, lived expertise, and rich knowledge systems.

Culture

Cultural competence, in medicine and public health, refers to understanding and attending to culturally diverse backgrounds of patients and providing culturally appropriate, person-centered care to all patients. The model of a "culturally competent" healthcare system has been defined as "one that acknowledges and incorporates—at all levels—the importance of culture, assessment of cross-cultural relations, vigilance toward the dynamics that result from cultural differences, expansion of cultural knowledge, and adaptation of services to meet culturally unique needs" (Betancourt et al., 2005, p. 201). As public health administrators have sought to address the mechanisms underpinning health disparities along racial and ethnic lines, public health initiatives have identified bias and poor cross-cultural communication between providers and their patients from racialized, minority, and immigrant populations as a cause of health disparities. To reverse these disparities, providers should learn about the backgrounds, worldviews, languages, and cultures of the diverse patient populations they served (Jongen, McCalman, and Bainbridge, 2018; Betancourt et al., 2003). The vision here is that culturally competent providers will support more people to access, use, and comply with medicine; in turn, patients will experience better health outcomes, and health disparities will lessen.

In service of cultural competence, several practices have become commonplace and, often, institutionally mandated. First, there are efforts to diversify in the healthcare profession at all levels. Not only does research suggest that patients from marginalized groups are more likely to trust a provider from the same group (Cooper-Patrick et al., 1999; Smedley et al., 2001; Cohen, Gabriel, and Terrell, 2002; Mansh, Garcia, and Lunn, 2015), but racial, ethnic, and language concordance between patient and provider has been shown to lead to better care and improved health outcomes for patients from marginalized groups (Greenwood et al., 2020; Snyder et al., 2023). The culture frame also attends to structural barriers that people from marginalized backgrounds face when trying to use healthcare. Accordingly, culture-based approaches aim to alleviate systemic barriers to healthcare (Betancourt et al., 2003; Betancourt et al., 2005). Provider training also has a prominent place in achieving culturally competent healthcare systems. The origins of cultural competency training in the US are traceable to early diversity training efforts following civil rights legislation in the 1960s (Anand and Winters, 2008). Today, common are trainings in cultural competence, cultural safety, cultural humility, and cultural intelligence and in overlapping areas including diversity training, antiracism training, and microaggression training (Shepherd, 2019). These trainings typically include educational initiatives aimed at teaching providers knowledge, tools, and skills that will help them understand and provide quality care to diverse patient populations. Trainings often focus on health beliefs, cultural and religious beliefs, language differences, and cultural norms that shape how different people might relate to medicine (Lekas, Pahl, and Fuller Lewis, 2020). While some cultural-competence trainings are based on content, other trainings have moved to a more process-based model that emphasizes listening and openness to individual patients, their concerns and beliefs, their values and priorities, and the contexts in which they seek healthcare (Betancourt et al., 2005). Helping to propel this latter direction, physicians and activists Melanie Tervalon and Jann Murray Garcia (1988) responded to the late twentieth-century embrace of cultural competency by advocating for a different, more critical approach, which they called cultural humility. Cultural humility is not predicated on the idea that one person can master another culture, as a body of content, but teaches providers to practice an openness to learning about others' backgrounds and contexts, self-reflexivity about one's own cultural positioning, and commitment to listening to and collaborating with patients.

As Tervalon and Garcia's intervention suggests, there have also been important critiques of culture as a frame to approach poor health outcomes and noncompliance. Despite the prevalence of culture-based training for healthcare professionals, there's little evidence that these trainings work in terms of increasing patient self-reported satisfaction with their care, improving health outcomes, or reducing health disparities (Lekas, Pahl, and Fuller Lewis, 2020; Jongen et al., 2018). Cultural trainings can reproduce simplistic and homogenous ideas about another culture; Stephan Shepherd (2018) has argued that many cultural-awareness workshops adopt a "museum approach" to another culture "whereby attendees are briefly exposed to a catalog of cultural artifacts and traditions" and then go on their way. Cultural competence trainings can risk stereotyping, othering, exoticizing, romanticizing, or stigmatizing patients in ways that further entrench racist attitudes and systems (Downing and Kowal, 2011). Cultural competence also leaves little room to consider intersectionality, the heterogeneity of culture, and the ways that different sociocultural and systemic conditions can intersect and shape patient experiences and outcomes. Rarely centered in trainings are the ways that trauma and ongoing racism can shape health beliefs and outcomes (Herring et al., 2013; Benjamin, 2013, pp. 39–44). Culture, like literacy, can rewrite structural problems as individual ones; the culture frame can atomize dissent into individual issues of cultural belief and difference.

Trust

Trust focuses on relationships between people and institutions. In the trust frame, it is less an individual's responsibility to find and trust the right information; rather, it is the responsibility of institutions—healthcare, public health, and the government—to operate such that people *can* trust them and follow their advice. Philosopher of science Maya Goldenberg, in her 2021 book *Vaccine Hesitancy: Public Trust, Expertise, and the War on Science,* argues that the popular understanding of vaccine hesitancy as a war on science is wrong and should be reframed as a crisis of trust. Goldenberg explains that "public trust hinges on the value set that influences scientific research [. . .] not only epistemic rigor but also equity and social responsibility" (p. 125), or, as Hausman (2022) rephrases: "you can have all the epistemic rigor in the world, but if I don't trust you, I won't believe your findings." Goldenberg identifies medical racism, social media, and the commercialization of science as phenomena that have corroded public trust in science and medicine. Thus, the solution to vaccine hesitancy and medical noncompliance more generally is not one that relies on connecting more people with good scientific information and medical resources; rather, solutions necessitate that institutions invest in the diverse populations they serve and thereby earn people's trust.

Others, though, have warned that trust, as a framework, focuses too much on relationships and individual feelings of good will, to the exclusion of policy and structural change. Sociologist Ruha Benjamin (2013) has argued that so much hand-wringing over trust and the reasons why people don't trust medicine and all it has to offer ignores the "elephant in the room"—that many racialized and marginalized people don't trust medicine because medicine, as an institution, has harmed and excluded them (p. 135). Benjamin is critical of public health, medical, and social-scientific approaches that invest so much energy into deciphering the reasons that different people don't trust science and scientific evidence, when the reasons should be obvious. Benjamin further critiques how the trust frame rewrites structural inequities into interpersonal problems. By naming the problem as distrust, the solution is in improved, interpersonal relations rather than structural change that accounts for histories of racism and discrimination and that invests in democratic and inclusive governance of science (pp. 135–141; p. 181).

Other scholars have identified limitations in how the trust frame explains noncompliance. First, the definition of *trust* itself is far from settled (Luhmann, 1979; Giddens, 1990), and yet the term is often used as if everyone shares a common understanding of what trust is and why it matters. Trust is often leveraged as a monolithic, all-or-nothing state (Hobson-West, 2007), as a "catch-all" category that blocks more granular insights (Leach and Fairhead, 2008, p. 29). Studies that engage people's perspectives on vaccination, for example, show that vaccine hesitancy can rarely be attributed wholly to distrust; many vaccine-hesitant parents do not resist all vaccines but selectively vaccinate, or vaccinate on spread-out schedules, or change their vaccination practices as their perceptions of their vulnerabilities, environments, and potential benefits shift (Wentzell and Racila, 2021; Hausman, 2017, pp. 298–299). Such findings are not commensurate with an explanation of vaccine hesitancy as caused by distrust of medicine and government. Further complicating the trust frame, distrust in some areas of medicine is often expected of responsible healthcare consumers. In contexts other than vaccination, there reigns a neoliberal expectation that good health citizens—especially if they are mothers—should approach medicine with a dose of skepticism, should do their own research, and should approach their providers as informed partners in their own health decision-making (Derkatch, 2022; Hausman, 2019, pp. 67–69; Jack, 2014, pp. 65–72; Reich, 2014). The neoliberal expectation that we all do our research and optimize our own health is bracketed in the trust frame, wherein distrust is positioned as a delinquent stance. Finally, the trust frame is also used differently and harmfully to explain vaccine dissent in the global South. Public health and health policy texts about vaccine hesitancy in the global North position vaccine hesitancy as a postmodern affliction, where the breakdown in trust is a symptom of modern persons' reflexive, spiraling anxieties about modern life and all its unknowns (Giddens, 1990). In the global South, distrust is attributed to people's premodern status; here, trust in institutions has *not yet been* established (Leach and Fairhead, 2008, p. 22). Such handlings of trust reify homogenizing notions of people in the global South as premodern, defined by superstition and unenlightened cultural beliefs.

The trust frame, like the literacy and culture frames, relies on a deficit approach to medical dissent. Health literacy is about winning over minds, and trust is about winning over hearts (Leach and Fairhead, 2008, p. 4). All three frames are grounded in an idea that the public lacks something (literacy, trust, shared cultural mores). In the trust frame, providers, institutions, and power structures may understandably make it hard for people, especially marginalized people, to trust the knowledge proffered by the same systems that have oppressed them. But medical knowledge itself is unproblematic. It is the stewards of the knowledge who need to do more social outreach and relationship repair to help ensure that more people can trust and use their expert knowledge, systems, and technologies. The following section explores how scholars in the humanities and social sciences have taken up another set of terms—*resistance, suspicion,* and *refusal*—to analyze medical dissent in ways that are not predetermined by a biomedical worldview and that theorize dissent as creative and productive.

Beyond a Medical Purview:
Resistance, Suspicion, and Refusal as Generative Dissent

Humanist and social-science research has advanced the concepts of resistance, suspicion, and refusal to frame medical dissent, to different degrees, as generative. Within these three frames, the purpose of studying dissent is not necessarily to achieve compliance. The aim is to listen to and learn from "no." Each concept, though, has a different bent. *Resistance* is oriented to noticing and learning from activist and coalition-building acts of dissent. *Suspicion* attends to the affective dimensions of dissent. *Refusal* is useful to label both an object of study (the "no") and a method of analysis (following the "no"); *refusal* implicates the researcher, too, in considerations of what is being refused and why. The following subsections engage each concept further.

Resistance

Resistance refers to a range of actions—protest, advocacy, disobedience, agitation, subversion, opposition—undertaken to actively oppose and critique medicine and healthcare. Resistance can take many different forms, from political activism against medical and pharmaceutical institutions to individual acts of disengagement. In the public sphere, health social movements and organized acts of resistance have challenged state, institutional, and cultural authorities about matters of health and medicine; resistive social movements challenge medical policy, public health policy and politics, medical research practices, the pharmaceutical industry, the authority of medical knowledge and expertise, and health-related inequities. Most recognizable is resistance advanced through public, organized protest and activism. The women's health movement in the 1970s and 1980s and AIDS/HIV activism, including the work of ACT UP, in the 1980s and 1990s are two widely studied sites of health resistance and activism; both have resulted in long-term changes in social attitudes about medicine, medical research, clinical practice, and the role of patients in healthcare. But healthcare resistance is enacted in many forms, such as advocacy for gender-affirming care (s. schuster, 2021), for access to reproductive healthcare (Kline, 2010), and for reproductive justice (Roberts, 1997; Kluchin, 2009). Health resistance may take the form of activism against health inequities—for example, much activism has arisen around experiences of environmental racism and its health effects (Brown, 2007; Alaimo, 2010). Other forms of activism have arisen around contested illnesses and illness experiences, especially chronic, poorly understood illnesses; individuals have formed biosocial groups around shared illness experiences and advocated for wider, medical recognition of their illness experiences (Brown, 2007; Dumes, 2020). During the COVID pandemic, there arose many competing health movements—groups arguing against masking and public health mandates, while others called for a greater sense of social responsibility and the need for ongoing public health safety measures.

Resistance also coheres outside of the public sphere, in individual decisions and daily actions and within communities. For example, rhetoricians and technical communication scholars have examined how resistance happens online, where individuals form their own digital communities to help each other navigate medical institutions, vet medical advice, learn from and exchange experiential knowledge, use medical knowledge in unsanctioned ways, and find interpersonal support and community as well as therapeutic guidance outside of medical encounters (Holladay, 2017; Edenfield, Holmes, and Colton, 2019; Pengilly, 2020). Across this small sampling of acts and types of resistance, though, there is the commonality that resistance is an intentional act of opposition. Resistance as a framework is therefore attuned to the political reasons that people opt out of, critique, protest, or build alternatives to medicine and medical care.

In scholarly spaces, feminist, Black feminist, disability studies, and queer theory scholars have led the way in studying resistance as the discursive and material strategies that subjugated groups have harnessed to challenge power. *Resistance* is a cornerstone of disability studies, a field that has critiqued and resisted the medicalization of disability. The medicalization of disability refers, broadly, to the pathologizing of disability and the normative medical drive to cure disabled people (Davis, 1995; Clare, 2017; Kafer, 2013). In *Feminist, Queer, Crip*, Alison Kafer (2013) describes biomedical narratives of disability as unfolding along "curative time," which frames cure as the only desirable future for disabled people. Eunjung Kim (2017) has situated biomedical, cure-based approaches to disability in the legacy of colonialism; Kim extends Kafer's argument to argue that a rehabilitated body becomes a sign of sovereign statehood under capitalism, for the colonized state was understood as a disabled body. A neutralized medical model of disability facilitates curative violence to work on many dimensions—the individual, the family, the community, the state, the ethno-nation-state—and to obscure violence committed in the name of a cure (Kim, 2017). Sayantani DasGupta has argued that the medical model of disability is enmeshed with capitalism; medical and cure-driven approaches to disability are aimed not at health but rather at keeping "those bodies perceived to be unproductive and/or nonnormative sequestered, controlled, diagnosed, and otherwise administered to by the medical profession" (2015, p. 123). These arguments help to show how resistance in health and medicine is wide-spanning and challenges foundational systems and normative structures. In response, disability, queer, Black feminist, feminist, and other health activists have analyzed, theorized, and cultivated resistance against medical approaches that identify and intervene in problems at the level of the individual body and thereby obscure structural and social determinants of health. These examples skim the surface of resistance in health and medicine, but they demonstrate that this term is useful to name the ways that groups and people, from positions of a relative lack of power, have challenged medicine's expertise and authority, medical research and clinical practice, and the entanglements of medicine, politics, and profit.

Suspicion

Charles (2022) developed the concept of suspicion from her ethnographic study of a global public health campaign for HPV vaccination in Barbados.[4] Charles began her study by considering Afro-Barbadian women who turned down HPV vaccines to be vaccine-hesitant but came to reject the term *vaccine hesitancy* as overdetermined by a biomedical perspective that preemptively defined hesitancy as a "delay or refusal purportedly rooted in ignorance" (p. 5). Drawing from the words of Afro-Barbadian mothers and young women targeted for vaccination, Charles theorizes suspicion as an "embodied affective intensity" that accrues at the intersections of harmful systems and histories. Suspicion is an "affective relation that circulates in the various socioeconomic, political, cultural, and historical formations that contextualize the vaccine." These systems include "growing assemblages of multinational pharmaceutical networks and the state, and longer transnational histories of slavery, capitalist extraction, and public health" (p. 13). Suspicion is about emotional intensities and gut feelings. It is sticky, contagious, elusive. It is something felt, and it circulates and accretes meaning and intensity over time. As an affective energy rather than a specific argument, suspicion directs attention away from the thing being refused—in Charles's study, the HPV vaccine—and toward the systems that produce suspicion. As an affective stance, suspicion eschews discourses of rationality versus irrationality, ignorance, and deficit. Instead, suspicion is useful for attending to the histories, systems, and everyday experiences that enshroud an ordinary object, like a vaccine, with risk and duplicity. Suspicion "reveals care's inequalities and political stakes"; in doing so, suspicion unsettles biomedical claims that the HPV vaccine is "*the* means to

---

4. Charles's study began when the HPV was introduced into Barbados in 2014 as part of a global effort to get 10- to 12-year-old girls in Barbados vaccinated. Public health officials attributed the program's lack of success—vaccination rates barely hit 20%—to Barbadian parents' ignorance, miseducation, and puritanical concerns about adolescent girls' sexuality. But, drawing on interviews, Charles pieced together a different story, one that insisted that low vaccination rates could not be disentangled from Barbadians' histories and experiences with colonial biopolitics and the surveillance and control of Black female sexuality from the period of slavery onward.

care and protection" and makes room for other forms of care (p. 15). To this end, Charles proposes a form of "radical care" defined as "outside colonial and scientific claims to objectivity and rationality, processes of pharmaceuticalization, neoliberal governmentality, and state-industry partnerships, all through which the HPV vaccine came to be realized" (p. 151). Suspicion is therefore a powerful concept for attending to the affective dimensions of vaccine decision-making. While we might debate whether claims about specific vaccine risks are right or wrong, these dimensions—right, wrong; fact, fiction; logical, illogical—are less applicable when trying to understand affect. And so, the discussion about vaccination must turn to the histories, assemblages, and experiences that sustain bad feelings—suspicion—beyond the binary of whether they are scientifically valid or not.

Refusal

Resistance and refusal cover much of the same terrain, but *refusal* is a distinct term useful to name dissent that is generative (Charles, 2022, pp. 10–12; Mcgranahan, 2016). Anthropologist Carole McGranahan (2016) has argued that refusal is a necessary term because it can be used to label acts that cannot be mapped onto a story of resistance and domination (p. 320). In this subsection, I stray from the focus on medical dissent to engage anthropologist Audra Simpson's work on the ethnographic refusal (2007, 2014, 2017), which has been formative in theorizing refusal. I then return to refusals in medicine and address how scholars of health and medicine have taken up Simpson's work.

Simpson theorized the ethnographic refusal in articles (2007, 2017) and *Mohawk Interruptus* (2014), an ethnography based on her research with the Mohawks of Kahnawà:ke. Simpson's ethnographic refusal derives from a specific exchange with an informant. During fieldwork, Simpson had been interviewing members of the Kahnawà:ke tribe to explore Kahnawà:ke understandings of Canadian rules for tribe membership. In one interview, Simpson asked an informant about Canadian membership rules, and the informant claimed that no one knew the rules of membership. Simpson, not only a researcher but also a member of the Kahnawà:ke herself, knew that this claim was not true; everyone who lived in the Kahnawà:ke community debated Canadian-imposed rules of membership (2014, p. 108). Simpson pushed her informant to say more. Still, the informant refused to change his answer (pp. 108–109). Why was her informant lying in such an obvious way? Simpson identified this exchange as an ethnographic refusal. The informant's refusal was a sign that Simpson, as the ethnographer, was no longer working to produce knowledge that was useful to her community, the Mohawks of Kahnawà:ke. Thus, the informant's nonanswer did not signify a failed interview; the refusal was an opening to end this line of inquiry and look elsewhere. "Enough," Simpson heard in the refusal, "was enough" (p. 111). The informant's refusal was not just a reorientation for this study but also a revisioning of what scholarship should do.

To this point, Indigenous scholars Eve Tuck and K. Wayne Yang (2014a; 2014b) have theorized refusal in social-science research as a move that researchers and research participants make to surface the processes of settler-colonial knowledge production and to disrupt colonial futurity. Beginning from the premise that research has been used to study, commodify, and speak for the subaltern, the authors argue that refusals, like the ones Simpson identifies and follows, redirect researchers away from the illusion of complete knowledge and "to ideas otherwise unacknowledged or unquestioned" (2014a, p. 225), to ways to "learn from and respect the wisdom and desires in the stories that we (over)hear, while refusing to portray/betray them to the spectacle of the settler colonial gaze" (p. 227), to "care and curiosity" (p. 227). "A methodology of refusal," the authors write, "regards limits on knowledge as productive, as indeed a good thing" (p. 233). Refusals are humanizing, for researchers most of all; refusals cleave an opening for researcher and researched to work together to make explicit the "metanarrative" of settler colonialism in knowledge production, what Tuck and Yang term "the code beneath the code," and to follow that refusal as "a starting place for other qualitative analyses and interpretations of data," which often involve refusing to study people and publish findings in academic venues (2014b, p. 812). Indeed, Simpson's encounter with refusal realigned Simpson's study away from questions about Kahnawà:ke understandings of tribal membership and to the questions "What am I revealing here and why? Where will this get us? Who benefits from this and why?" (2014, p. 111).

Simpson's ethnographic refusal, as well as Tuck and Yang's development of Simpson's ethnographic refusal, is specifically a form of Indigenous refusal, but the ethnographic refusal has been taken up in other contexts, including studies of medical dissent. Benjamin (2016) built on Simpson's work to theorize the informed refusal in her research on "biodefection," defined as nonparticipation in common medical institutions, behaviors, and logics. Informed refusal rejects the assumption built into informed consent that people, if given accurate and understandable information, will consent to medical plans. By suggesting that refusal, like consent, can be informed, Benjamin's work asks: What kind of information, experience, and context informs this refusal? When does refusal make sense? Why doesn't medicine work well for everyone? "An informed refusal," Benjamin explains, "is seeded with a vision of what can and should be, and not only a critique of what is" (p. 970). Medical anthropologist Elisa Sobo has also built on Simpson's work to theorize refusals as affiliative. For Sobo, refusal, unlike resistance, is not always an "act of standing against" (2016, p. 342); sometimes, refusal is an act of opting in. To illustrate this type of refusal, Sobo turned to her ethnographic study of a Waldorf school, a school wherein parents secured personal belief exemptions to vaccination at much higher rates than in other schools. In this Waldorf school, vaccine refusal was the norm. Thus, the decision to not vaccinate was not so much a resistance against vaccination or against public health. Vaccine refusal was a prosocial opting *into* the Waldorf community. This refusal was motivated by a desire to belong. Here, refusal was a "communion-centered," "future-oriented" act, a "promise to one's child of future good health and a vow to one's associates of continual association" (p. 347). Refusal was a move to find, build, and signal commitment to community. As such, we might listen for the types of communities, relationships, and modes of belonging that medical refusal makes possible.

Rhetorical Refusal

Resistance, suspicion, and refusal are explanatory frames that respond to medical dissent not necessarily as a medical problem but as an opening to practice care, medicine, illness, and health otherwise. Rhetorical refusal, too, engages dissent as an informed and generative act as well as a rhetorical one. This section begins with three glimpses of rhetorical refusal in action. These fragments provide examples of rhetorical refusal, and the remainder of this section defines rhetorical refusal and its scope and stakes.

Ayaan was a student in Midnimo's inaugural health literacy course, which was developed by and for Somali women. One objective of the course was that students would learn that the MMR vaccine does not cause autism, and that autism is a neurodevelopmental disability. Ayaan had two children who had been diagnosed with microcephaly; she told me that she was eager to learn more about healthcare. Ayaan did well on the course's quizzes, and yet Ayaan continued to describe her two children as having autism. When I asked Ayaan why she referred to her children as having autism despite their diagnoses of microcephaly, she told me that autism was "our community's sickness." Autism, she explained, was a sickness that Somali children encountered in the US. The health literacy course, it appeared, had not changed Ayaan's notion that autism, for Somali children, was a unique, Western illness. The health literacy course-evaluation forms labeled Ayaan's use of "autism" as an error, one that called for more health education. But, in chapter 1, I argue that Ayaan's and fellow students' misuses of medical terms were rhetorical refusals that called attention to exigences of rhetorical refusal, exigences that shaped their everyday lives, even as they were elided and dismissed in health literacy frameworks.

In an interview about her experience of the 2017 measles outbreak, Kowsar told me that she was tired of being told that she didn't understand science. Yes, she hadn't vaccinated her children with the MMR vaccine. But it wasn't because she thought there was some government plot or mercury in the vaccine. Kowsar asked, had I considered that Somali refugees had likely received extra doses of a measles vaccine? Maybe one kind of vaccine as a child in Somalia, another in a refugee camp, then another one in the US. Could I tell her what studies examined the effects of extra shots? And then the generational effects down the line? I could tell her that WHO and CDC had stated that multiple rounds of vaccination did not pose dangers to refugees. But I didn't have an answer when Kowsar asked why, if public health could not trust mothers about their children's vaccine histories without papers, she should believe public health policies had refugees' health interests at heart. Healthcare, Kowsar insisted, was not designed for people like her.

One afternoon, when I was observing community health workers and Somali mothers working together to complete applications for state disability services, I watched Nimo, a Somali mother, work through a series of questions that asked if her child struggled to meet "age-appropriate milestones," such as dressing and toileting. Nimo stopped midway through, turned over the application, and told her collaborating community health worker a story about her son Isse. She described shared jokes in the family. She spoke of his favorite words and his beloved trucks. That afternoon, Nimo completed the application on behalf of her young son, but she never submitted her paperwork to the state. Her departure from the grant program was recorded as a failure in Midnimo's outcomes assessments. But in chapter 3, I read Nimo's unsubmitted application as a rhetorical refusal, oriented toward protection and brimming with futurity.

Rhetorical refusal is a communicative act of dissent against or disengagement from institutional knowledge and practices. Rhetorical refusal begins from the premise that there can be significance to dissent, that dissent can be rhetorical, participatory, and generative. Rhetorical refusal situates dissent outside of the compliance/noncompliance binary, outside of the drive to convert noncompliance into compliance, and outside of the debate about whether dissent is aligned with or against science and scientific evidence. Rarely, Gouge (2018) has argued, is noncompliance studied as a "complex issue that rhetoricians might address" (p. 115); instead, questions of noncompliance bounce back and forth within the frames of literacy, culture, and trust, remaining limited to considerations of persuasion, information delivery, and the role of expertise. Also writing about the unexamined dimensions of noncompliance in medicine, rhetorician Judy Z. Segal (2005) has argued that noncompliance "does not need to be obsessively measured, and it does not, as a concept, need to be rijigged out of existence. The actions of patients need to be studied not mechanistically but with an appropriately complex theory of human persuasion and human judgment: a theory of rhetoric" (p. 151).

Rhetorical refusal considers what contexts inform dissent and what futures dissent makes possible. Rhetorical refusal encompasses a range of modes, including speaking and writing as well as not writing, deferring writing, being silent, using one's body, caring for another's body, making a mistake, listening, translating, mistranslating, leaving, looking away, and quitting. In this book, I address rhetorical refusals articulated through alternative and wrong vocabularies (chapter 1); embodied nonaction (chapter 2); mistakes, absences, and silences in institutional documentation (chapter 3); and everyday practices of care (chapter 4). Across these chapters, rhetorical refusals are articulated in many ways, such as a silence in response to a healthcare provider's question, a missed well-child visit, an unsigned disability evaluation, or a blank space on a medical intake form. These are acts that might be read as nonrhetorical, as outside of the parameters of argument, intentional communication, and rhetoricity. These acts might not seem to have much to do with language, argument, speakers, audiences, or persuasion—the bread and butter of rhetoric. But these lapses and blank spaces, these departures and domestic practices are rhetorical. Seemingly nonrhetorical modes of dissent are vital for rhetors communicating from the margins, for rhetors for whom publicity is not always available or safe, as I explain more in this section. Rhetorical refusal, as a concept, demarcates dissent communicated by marginalized rhetors to create space apart from institutional knowledge, norms, and practices. Rhetorical refusals make meaning, disrupt flows of power, carve space apart from institutional and dominant worldviews, signal to and cohere publics. Rhetorical refusals protect, argue, and circulate possibilities.

A useful starting place to approach the rhetoricity of rhetorical refusal is rhetorician and disability scholar Jay Dolmage's definition of rhetoric as "the strategic study of the circulation of power through communication" (2014, p. 3). This definition does not center an individual rhetor's intention and discrete communicative act; instead, rhetoric is about flux and movements of meaning, power, and agency. "Rhetoric," rhetorician and queer disability theorist J. Logan Smilges (2022) has written by way of definition, "is less about the linear exchange of information from a single rhetor to an audience and more about the production of meaning between and among living, breathing, and moving things and people" (p. 8). Rhetorical refusals emanate rhetoricity in these matrices of meaning, where an incomplete document, a missed vaccination, an alternative use of a medical term can all push against power relations, interrupt the status quo, and breach new futures. Rhetorical refusal, as a concept, helps illuminate the stakes of attending to such seemingly nonrhetorical, seemingly apolitical, seemingly nonagentive acts as rhetorical, political, and agentive.

Why read silences, absences, blank pages, mistakes, and withdrawals as rhetorical? Doing so is crucial to study rhetoric in spaces where power is asymmetrical. When power is asymmetrical, traditional rhetorical action—writing, speaking—is not universally possible, accessible, and safe. Rhetoricians Jennell Johnson and Krista Kennedy (2020) have challenged the assumption that visibility—which encompasses representation, voice, being seen and heard—is a good, empowering thing, essential to political action and social change. "In visibility politics," Johnson and Kennedy write, "rhetorical agency and political action are understood as tightly interlinked," but this model does not account for the risks and harms that visibility can bring to marginalized persons. The authors continue,

> To be visible, especially as a person from a marginalized community, is to "summon surveillance and the law" (Phelan, 6). Although invisibility may be the result of oppression (as people in the dominant population choose not to "see" or "show" those who don't fit the norm), "forced visibility" can also lead to surveillance, doxing, deportation, firing, and even violence or death. (p. 162)

Further, when marginalized rhetors do speak, there is no guarantee that their voices will be heard. Philosopher Miranda Fricker (2007) developed the terms *epistemic marginalization* and *testimonial injustice* to account for the ways that marginalized people are denied the role of "epistemic agent" and excluded from the work of creating knowledge and of communicating with credibility and expertise (refer also to Vinson, 2017; Britt, 2018; Harper, 2021). Rhetorician M. Remi Yergeau (2018) has argued that some persons (in Yergeau's study, autistic persons) "can never reach rhetoricity" as they are rendered "residual, lesser, and inhuman" and suspended in "half-rhetoricity" or "demi-rhetoricity," which "functions effectually as non-rhetoricity" (p. 46). Accounting for the rhetoricity granted to some subjects and withheld from others, rhetorician Christa Teston, also drawing on Yergeau's concept of rhetoricity, has defined rhetoric as a "normative term that discriminates as much as it describes" (2024, p. 8).

Rhetorician Mary Lay (2000) has shown that a rhetor's available rhetorical tools are contingent on "the degree of authority one's knowledge carries" (p. 22). Some people are granted the epistemic and rhetorical privilege of being "knowers," or "experts whose judgment and knowledge count" (p. 22). Others are not. Lay's work shows that, in health-related spaces, anyone who speaks from a nonmedical vantage point—for example, from their own experience or from an alternative system of understanding the body and health—is rhetorically disadvantaged. This rhetorical diminishment is compounded for those speaking from positions of marginalization, as is the case for Somali American mothers, who are multiply marginalized in the US by race, ethnicity, religion, gender, and, often, class and language backgrounds. Rhetorician Kimberly Harper (2021) has argued that rhetorical scholars too often assume that speakers always have agency, by virtue of being speakers, and thereby overlook how "a group of people or individuals can have an ethos that is created and managed by outside forces" (p. 232). Harper depicts how Black women in the US speak from positions of constrained agency as their ethos is overdetermined by powerful tropes and preset rhetorical subjectivities, including those of "breeder, mammy, matriarch, jezebel, welfare queen, pregnant drug addict, and teen mother" (p. 233; refer also to Collins, 1990). Somali American mothers' voices, too, are overdetermined, with narratives of illiteracy, trauma, and tragedy, such that medical professionals often read Somali American mothers' noncompliant actions as unfortunate results of illiteracy and fear and not as intentional, strategic, and generative arguments.

Lay (2000) has asked, in response to this uneven, power-pocked terrain of public discourse, "how rhetors who seem less powerful than their opposition negotiate the common reality, the knowledge systems, within any particular discourse community they join or argue against" (p. 22). This inquiry remains pressing for rhetorical scholarship and action; almost twenty years later, rhetorician Shui-yin Sharon Yam (2019), in her study on citizenship in Hong Kong, posed similar questions: "What rhetorical conditions and tactics can marginalized subjects create and deploy in order to motivate those at a relative position of power to engage with them as equal interlocutors whose interests overlap and could redefine theirs?" and "What strategies can marginalized subjects deploy to be recognized on their own terms, rather than in a way that subsumes difference and reinforces the oppressive logic of the existing structure?" (p. 2). Rhetorical refusal is one way that rhetors who speak—or who do not speak—from positions of epistemic marginalization and testimonial injustice (Fricker, 2007) or compromised *ethos* (Harper, 2021) participate in institutional systems and public discourses wherein power is uneven and consolidated to the experts, the "knowers" (Lay, 2000), the institutional insiders, the powerful. Rhetorical refusal is one vital strategy that marginalized subjects create to tell their stories; insist on their interests and the validity of their experiences, knowledges, and concerns; protect themselves; and build coalitions toward different futures.

When it comes to expanding notions of rhetoric, rhetorical agency, and rhetorical action by attending to the rhetoricity of acts outside of speaking and writing, the stakes are high. Doing so is critical to rhetoric's ability to listen to and learn from marginalized rhetors. Rhetorical refusal joins rhetorical scholarship that has theorized the rhetoricity of seemingly passive or nonrhetorical modes of meaning-making and argumentation, including silence (Glenn, 2004; Smilges, 2022); rhetorical listening (Ratcliffe, 2005); invisibility (Johnson and Kennedy, 2020); rhetorical quieting (Smilges, 2022); participatory nonuse (Green, 2021); closetedness (Cox, 2019); nondisclosure (Kerschbaum, 2014); and touch (Dolmage, 2014; Walters, 2014). In these studies, scholars have approached what may seem to be nonrhetorical actions, or even a lack of action, as agentive, meaningful, and rhetorical. Smilges's (2022) work on queer silence offers a theoretical frame to approach the seemingly nonrhetorical; Smilges introduces queer silence as a concept that severs the link between agency and traditional speech or writing (p. 32) and, in turn, situates rhetoricians to "use a wider net to reveal the meaning-making strategies enacted by minoritarian populations to defend themselves against dominant discourses" (p. 8). To do so, rhetoricians should turn "away from what people are saying to what they aren't, away from who is speaking to who is remaining silent, and away from speech entirely toward the ways silence has been signifying all along" (p. 9). By studying acts like silence as rhetorical, rhetoricians can attend to the "surprising potentialities of silence to generate meaning from absence and the ways people on the margins of society tap into these potentialities in order to build community, navigate hostile spaces, and resist forms of institutional and state sponsored violence" (p. 4). In this book, I theorize rhetorical refusal as a concept that can continue the work of weaving "a wider net to reveal the meaning-making strategies" (p. 8). In health and medicine, rhetorical refusals are often misread as errors, passivity, or routines, but rhetorical refusal is a tool for recognizing these under-the-radar acts as rhetorical and meaningful. Rhetorical refusal is a concept useful for naming and listening to seemingly nonrhetorical acts as acts of communicative dissent and disengagement. Within medical frames and worldviews, these acts are often automatically defined as errors, the symptoms of deficient health literacy, and results of access barriers. Rhetorical refusal offers a way to reframe seeming mistakes, absences, nonuse, and nonparticipation as intentional resistance, ingroup protection, and participatory stances taken in commitment to different futures.

Rhetorical refusal provides infrastructure to listen to dissent as limned with meaning and possibility. In the chapters to come, I show that rhetorical refusals can be analyzed in three parts: the refusal, its fertile ground, and its futurity or arc. Rhetorical refusal is grounded in a discrete act—a silence, a statement, a blank application, an unfilled prescription. But a rhetorical refusal harkens back to lived contexts, histories, and logics, to the fertile ground that makes dissent logical, safe, or necessary. In mainstream public discourses, refusal's fertile ground is often misread as a lack of medical knowledge, a lack of scientific literacy, remediable by communicating accurate and tailored information to marginalized groups. Rhetorical refusal, as a concept, allows silences, mistakes, care practices, nonscientific practices, and absences to tell different stories. Rhetorical refusal orients listeners to dissent's historical, socially embedded, structural, and often bracketed contexts. Rhetorical refusal insists on exigences of dissent that break out of dominant frames and logics of dissent in which dissent is regarded as a problem of individual belief. Thirdly, rhetorical refusal also arcs toward different futures that open in lieu of the institutionally expected course of action.

Analyzing rhetorical refusals with attention to their arcs is an analytical strategy to engage Tuck and Yang's (2014a) argument that the generativity of refusal is a critical departure from social science research's peddling of "pain narratives," which "bemoan the food deserts, but forget to see the food innovations; they lament the concrete jungles and miss the roses and the tobacco from concrete"; refusal-informed research

> does not deny the experience of tragedy, trauma, and pain, but positions the knowing derived from such experiences as wise. This is not about seeing the bright side of hard times, or even believing that everything happens for a reason. Utilizing a desire-based framework [instead of a damage-focused one] is about working inside a more complex and dynamic understanding of what one, or a community, comes to know in (a) lived life. (p. 231)

This orientation to the positive productivity of refusal—which Tuck and Yang theorize as entwined with experiential knowledge—directs focus to what futures saying "no" opens up after dissenters refuse what, they are told, is the only right decision. In the context of refusals in health and medicine specifically, listening to dissent as a "rhetorically productive phenomenon" aims not just to understand noncompliance, dissent, and divergence more fully but to support better care, care that is not just medically sound but that responds to people's contexts, constraints, communities, values, and hopes (Gouge, 2018, p. 116). Listening to, rather than immediately correcting, dissent opens space to ask, "What kind of ethical action, what kind of care responses might divergence persuade?" (Gouge, 2018, p. 132). Listening to a rhetorical refusal involves identifying the refusal, following the refusal back to its fertile ground, and following the refusal forward to the futures it makes possible. Rhetorical refusal is therefore a concept useful for following the rhetorical ways that those outside of power participate in public discourse, form coalitions apart from the dominant public, and make space for different futures. In the following chapters, I develop this concept of rhetorical refusal by following participating Somali American parents' rhetorical refusals in spaces of healthcare, public health, health literacy education, social services, and the home.

The Study, Site, and Methods

This book is informed by twelve months of ethnographic fieldwork conducted in partnership with Midnimo, a Somali-run and Somali-serving women's health center in Minneapolis, Minnesota. Prior to this study, I had worked with Midnimo for two years as an English language literacy teacher. I was also a rhetorician who studied health and medicine and conducted qualitative research. As I worked more at Midnimo, Midnimo's executive director, Malyun, and I began to discuss collaborating on Midnimo's back-burner research agenda. Malyun aimed for Midnimo to develop its own research office that would support scholarship informed by the concerns of Midnimo's clients, Somali women in Minnesota. Our collaboration started small. We designed an internal study to assess the center's planned health literacy course. This internal study, however, was disrupted by the 2017 measles outbreak. With the measles outbreak, priorities shifted, and new questions proliferated. Midnimo partnered with public health offices and social-service agencies to deliver targeted health interventions to Somali Minnesotans; research priorities, as well, shifted to address how these interventions were working.

This study started with a crisis, the 2017 measles outbreak. The first part of the study focused on the measles outbreak and gathered stories from Somali parents, healthcare workers, and public health professionals about their outbreak experiences. The goal was to understand how Somali Minnesotans had responded to public health interventions during and following the outbreak. Next, the study shifted to follow autism interventions that were deployed as responses to the outbreak. After the outbreak, Midnimo was inundated with collaboration requests from state actors, who were newly invigorated to make inroads with Somali Minnesotan communities. Midnimo accepted private grant funding to launch its homegrown health literacy course, designed by and for Somali women. As a research partner, I observed the classes and co-conducted interviews and pre- and post-tests with participants to assess students' learning and self-reported experiences. In the wake of the outbreak, Midnimo also partnered with a county social-service department to administer short-term grants to families with children with autism. I studied how the grant process unfolded through artifact-based interviews, qualitative interviews, and field observations. The grant initiative, however, was largely unsuccessful, and many of the applicants left the program. A group of participants turned to naturopaths and microbiome-based care. Accordingly, this study moved to cover microbiome-informed autism care. This part of the study was informed by participants' visits with naturopaths and by stories about how microbiome theories of autism changed their approaches to care, illness, and health.

These four sites—health literacy class (chapter 1), the measles outbreak (chapter 2), social-service programming (chapter 3), and microbiome care (chapter 4)—make up the four spaces that anchor this study. At these sites, I conducted observations, qualitative interviews, and document-based interviews.[5] My field notes and interviews came primarily from the following interactions:

- autism support-group meetings
- autism workshops
- health literacy classes
- disability social-service workshops

---

5. These include the following:
- participatory observations (204 hours, concentrated mainly in support group meetings, health literacy classes, autism workshops, social-service meetings and visits, healthcare appointments, and time at family homes);
- qualitative interviews (79 interviews with 39 Somali parents, 10 community health workers, 3 Midnimo staff, 10 public health professionals, 8 healthcare providers, and 10 social-service professionals); and
- artifact-based interviews (79 interviews for 4 different documents with Somali parents (30), community health workers (30), medical professionals (3) and social-service professionals (16).

- case management meetings
- healthcare appointments
- community events
- internal meetings between social-service organizations and Midnimo staff
- Midnimo staff meetings
- public, social-service outreach programs and events
- community of practice meetings (meetings during which different stakeholders came together to talk about ways to expand autism resources to different communities and individuals)

While these sites encompass most interactions that informed my notes and interviews, not all of the stories reported in these pages come from one of these sites. As this study went on, my role expanded and blurred. I was not only taking notes as the resident researcher, but I was also writing Midnimo grant applications, helping stock food pantries, gathering in conference rooms for baby showers and graduation parties; I was driving all around town with Midnimo community health workers, setting up booths at summer festivals, reviewing younger siblings' college application essays, and spending time with the children whose parents I was interviewing. As participants' negotiations of health, illness, disability, and resources webbed far outside Midnimo, so, too, did my observations take me beyond the Midnimo's orange brick walls and temporary cubicles. I was spending time in participants' homes and neighborhood parks; I attended doctor appointments, conferences with educators, and caseworker sessions. These encounters, as well as the interactions listed above, inform the stories engaged in the chapters to come.

Across these sites, I was a participant observer; I went to meetings, events, classes, workshops, clinics, and homes as a researcher. Participants allowed me to take field notes with the goal of one day publishing the anonymized material. In addition to observations, I conducted qualitative interviews and document-based interviews with participants. The document-based interviews focused on the autism grant documentation that Somali American parents had to complete on behalf of their children and that county social-service staff evaluated. I conducted qualitative interviews throughout the study and with Somali parents, Midnimo staff, community health workers, public health personnel, healthcare providers, social-service staff, and naturopaths.

Lastly, this study's data collection included text-based analysis. I collected and analyzed news coverage, public health literature, medical literature, popular science and health writing, and disability-related outreach and documentation. These written texts shaped the rhetorical contexts in which Somali American parents advanced rhetorical refusals. To account for these public, institutional, and recorded discourses, each of the chapters opens with an account of the mainstream stories of each event; these are stories published in the mainstream media or documented by state institutions, such as public health. Each chapter then engages participants' stories. This approach is informed by rhetorician Aja Y. Martinez's (2020) methodology of counterstory, a narrative methodology geared to "telling stories by people whose experiences are not often told" (p. 6). In each chapter, the examination of mainstream, published discourses documents the "stock story" of a particular event, a story told by dominant groups until that story is "canonized or normalized" into "reality," such that all other versions are rendered "not credible" (2014, p. 36).[6] Somali American participants' refusals—silences, withdrawals, absences, mistakes, care practices—coupled with stories shared in interviews, weave into counterstories, "stories that disrupt the erasures embedded in standardized majoritarian methodologies" (or, in this case, narratives) (Martinez, 2020, p. 3). In each chapter, I approach rhetorical refusal as a mode of participating meaningfully in powerful, expert discourses—discourses in which Somali American parents did not have much access to ethos (Harper, 2021) or status as "knowers" (Lay, 2000). Rhetorical refusals happen in many contexts outside of the ones engaged in this study, and it is my goal that the analysis in this book will help others identify rhetorical refusals, recognize the exigences that engender rhetorical refusals, and follow refusals to the futures they work toward.

Throughout data collection and analysis, I practiced a "purposefully neutral stance toward vaccination" and other topics in science and medicine (Hausman et al., 2020, p. 249). Hausman (2019) has described the maintenance of a neutral stance as a "radical alienation from claims about scientific reasoning and scientific truth" (p. 236). As the chapters demonstrate, I do not classify participants' claims in terms of their scientific accuracy. That's because my goal is not to assess the veracity of participants' specific health-related claims but to inhabit participants' worldviews, the health logics and social histories that support specific claims.[7] I analyzed data by considering claims made by participants as embedded in their own worlds and shaped by material, sociopolitical, and historical contexts. Doing so was key to listening to the intricate arguments participants were making and to the ways that specific health decisions linked up to broader health beliefs and historical and social contexts (Lawrence, Hausman, and Dannenberg, 2014, p. 129). This

---

6. Martinez is engaging CRT (critical race theory) scholar Richard Delgado's work on stock stories.

7. Refer to Ratcliffe (2005) for a discussion of how rhetorical listening orients rhetoricians to hear logics rather than claims (pp. 32–33). I discuss rhetorical listening in terms of claims and logics in chapter 4.

stance brought refusal's stakes, contexts, and imagined futures into sharper relief. For these reasons, this book isn't *about* vaccines. This book is not *about* autism. I write about each term—*vaccination, health, autism, microbiome, community sickness*—as it functions within the worlds of participants and not as each term might be understood in other, external discourses. This book follows how certain terms, often terms with scientific, medical, and activist reverberations, including *vaccines* and *autism,* cohere rhetorical meaning and exert material influence within specific communities and in response to specific exigences.

This neutral stance was important to my analysis, but this stance does not mean that I was a neutral researcher. Necessarily, the data I collected and my interpretations are shaped by my own subjectivity and life experiences. As technical communication scholars Natasha Jones, Kristin Moore, and Rebecca Walton (2016) have explained, for all researchers, the "positionality, privilege, and power [. . .] inarguably affect and co-construct the ways in which people engage with identity markers such as race, ethnicity, gender, sexuality, ableness, religion, and class" (p. 225). Technical communication scholar Godwin Agboka (2013) has shown that reflection on one's own positionality as a researcher is key to rigorous and ethical research especially where imbalances of power are pronounced. My position as an outsider within Midnimo and as a white, US-born, English-speaking, able-bodied researcher who worked for a research university shaped my role and perspective in this project. Importantly, my position separated me from the stakes most pressing to Somali American participants. I could, when I wanted or needed, turn away from the life-absorbing experiences I recount in these pages, experiences of parents vying, day in and day out, to navigate complex systems, to weather personal discrimination and structural marginalization, to support their children within unfamiliar medical matrices, and to make decisions without even the flimsiest of safety nets. I immersed myself in these stories and worked alongside participants for local change, but I would never feel the worries weighing on my own chest, making me feel like I couldn't breathe, the way I've felt when the sanguinity of one of my own children has flitted from a given to a question. Too, many of the medical and public health models of health that excluded or harmed Somali American families have insulated me from risk, eased my access to medicine, and fostered my and my children's health. As a result, the stories recounted here are always partial. I hope that this practice of reflexivity, as Agboka (2013) theorized, has worked to keep the focus in this book's research approach on my commitment to listen, document honestly, and analyze scrupulously. This book aims to follow participants' leads, to work closely with participants and attune the research study to their expertise, and to build theory from participants' experiences.

About Autism

In the previous section, I wrote that this book is not about autism. And yet the word *autism* appears on almost every page. I want to take a few moments in this section to discuss the rhetorical uses of *autism* throughout these pages and to warn readers that some sources—participants, popular texts, and scientific articles—refer to autism in ableist and offensive ways. I'll start with the statement that this book is not about autism. This book is about dissent and refusal in medicine. Why do people refuse medicine? Why doesn't medicine work for everyone, even when the science is there to say it should? In exploring these questions with Somali partners and participants, autism came up in nearly every interview. Also in almost every interview, *autism* emerged as a rhetorical, flexible term, one used with many different meanings, by different rhetors, for different purposes, and within different epistemologies. Most often, Somali American parents used *autism* not as a name for a medical diagnosis and not to refer to a specific disability or to a specific form of neurodiversity. Somali American parents used autism as a social and political category useful to claim rhetorical space and compel collective action. This is an argument I build throughout the chapters, but to explain in brief: participants used autism as a trope to speak about health disparities and their day-to-day experiences of structural vulnerability to health risks. But why, readers might ask, use the term *autism*, a word that already has a specific meaning? Because *autism* retained its resonance as a scientific and biomedical term, participants used the term and its medical vocabulary to make more credible claims to institutions that had historically ignored their experiences and epistemologies of sickness. Put differently, people listened when Somali Minnesotans talked about autism. Accordingly, some Somali American participants used medical language and the language of biomedical diagnostics to occupy new subject positions, gain the attention of new audiences, harness rhetorical power, and get results. But this means that when participants spoke about autism as a political and social category, they often were not speaking about autism as it might relate to specific people, as a kind of neurodiversity. Helpful here is disability activist Simi Linton's work to redefine disability from a medical category into a social and political category. In Linton's words:

> When disability is redefined as a social/political category, people with a variety of conditions are identified as people with disabilities or disabled people, a group bound by common social and political experiences. These designations, as reclaimed by the community, are used to identify us as a constituency, to serve our needs for unity and identity, and to function as a basis for political activism (1998, p. 225).

Somali American parents often used the word *autism* and its associated vocabulary to refer not to a set of symptoms but to a "group bound by common social and political experiences." That is also why parents who were told their children had illnesses or disabilities that were not autism continued to identify with the label *autism*—it was a relevant social and political category, and one that could cohere groups and compel action. This is why, too, parents used the terms *autism* and *community sickness* interchangeably. In the chapters to follow, I explain how Somali American parents insisted on the ways that not just disability but race, ethnicity, religion, and histories of migration intersected with disability and were core to seeing and acting on autism as a sociopolitical category.

But participants did not always use autism in these ways, as a social and political category to compel collective action. As readers will see, some participants—Somali American parents, healthcare professionals, and service providers—did use *autism* to refer to an individual deficiency, a harmful and ableist stance. Some participating parents described autism as a loss. Mothers who felt that their children developed autism after a specific vaccination described seeing a light go out behind a child's eyes, described their child losing their ability to speak. Other parents described autism as something to fear and warned fellow parents not to vaccinate, lest they increase their own children's risk of developing autism. In my observations, therapists, community health works, and social service professionals often advised pursuing applied behavioral therapy (ABA), which many autistic adults and advocates have shown to be an abusive, harmful practice. Too, several of the written texts analyzed in these chapters advance ableist worldviews. Chapter 2 analyzes antivaccination discourses, which are notorious for advancing ableist and deeply harmful notions about autism. Antivaccination discourses often frame autistic children as the binary inverse of "normal" children and describe autism as a tragic diagnosis, one to be avoided at all costs. Autism is used to signify the risk of pollution and damage that can result from vaccines. "In these disabling discourses," historian Traci Brynne Voyles has argued, autism "is the relational inverse of the unpolluted body, a threat and a specter of difference" (2020). In chapter 3, participating naturopaths and collected texts about the human microbiome sometimes advance ableist notions about autism. Some microbiome experts and writers have categorized autism as a pathology of an unbalanced microbiome, have labeled so-called autistic behaviors as undesirable, and have prescribed probiotic cures to resolve these behaviors.

So, no, this book is not about autism. It is about clashing epistemologies and the rhetorical work that goes into refusing medical worldviews from a position of marginalization. But there's no avoiding that autism is often at the crosshairs of competing epistemologies and their attendant discourses.

There's no avoiding, too, that participants and texts sometimes advance ableist notions about autism and disability. And there's no avoiding that behind these stories, behind these rhetorical uses of autism, behind the leveraging of autism for much-needed rhetorical action, are the children on whose behalf participants spoke, acted, and refused. These children and their stories and voices are not a part of this book, but I want to acknowledge them and their indelible lives and interiorities. It is my hope that rhetorical refusal, particularly in its ability to surface expert and normative discourses and to voice yet-unimagined futures, can contribute to the work of breaking down these ableist structures.

Review of the Chapters

Chapter 1, "Welcome to Health Class: Community Sickness as Rhetorical Refusal's Fertile Ground," follows Midnimo's inaugural health literacy course. Chapter 1 begins in the classroom. This chapter charts how the homegrown course unfolded and focuses on the rhetorical, technical, and interpretive work that community health educators undertook to teach a medical discourse of autism. The chapter then shifts to the students, Somali American mothers. Here, the chapter focuses on a seeming contradiction: students scored well on their health literacy tests, but they also continued to use the term *community sickness* to refer to autism and continued to describe autism as a Western illness, unique to Somalis in diaspora. One way to interpret these misuses of autism-related vocabularies is as mistakes and signs that students' health literacy remains lacking. But I argue otherwise. Somali American students continued to use the term *community sickness* in intentional, precise ways. Parents used the discourses of community sickness to explain, tell stories about, and work toward solutions that related not to autism as an individual, medical problem but to the accretive ways that dislocation, loss, migration, racism, racialized surveillance, and structural precarity sickened them. For these reasons, the language of community sickness vividly depicts the fertile ground that seeded Somali participants' protective and participatory acts of dissent. Somali American students' uses of *community sickness* depict an important dimension of rhetorical refusal: rhetorical refusals do not always make activist arguments but sometimes work as affiliative rhetorical tools useful to cohere their own publics and to provide protection and care. The vocabulary of community sickness was one way that Somali mothers found and cared for one another.

Chapter 2, "Outbreak: Vaccine Dissent as Embodied Rhetorical Refusal," tells the less-heard stories of Somali American parents' vaccine decisions before, during, and after the 2017 measles outbreak. The first part of this chapter analyzes mainstream news media and public health accounts of the outbreak; these accounts tell a consistent story in which Somali Minnesotans were victims of targeted antivaccination campaigns. The second part of the chapter engages the voices of Somali parents who experienced the outbreak. Parents claimed and enacted forms of agency that news and public health narratives foreclosed for them. Parents' outbreak stories illustrate lived experiences of exclusion from the production of medical knowledge and the benefits of medical progress. Somali American parents' vaccine decision-making is therefore an important example of what happens when the herd we are told to protect becomes glaringly inequitable, when it's obvious that some members of the herd are asked to take on disproportionate risks while other members enjoy the most benefits. Navigating these fractured publics of public health, Somali American parents enacted rhetorical refusal through embodied nonaction, that is, selective nonvaccination. Participants' selective vaccine refusals are constrained and embodied acts of resistance and generative openings to collaboratively reenvision healthcare relationships, the structure of clinical trials and the evidence they produce, and the tenets of what counts as a healthy community. Read as rhetorical refusal, parents' vaccine refusals situate migration, racialization, and structural marginalization not just as experiences that mark a population but as important sites for contesting scientific knowledge and for forging new insights. For these reasons, there is epistemic value—not just symbolic significance—to rhetorical refusal; rhetorical refusal can, potentially, collaborate with and improve science and medical practice.

Chapter 3, "Writing to the State: Mistakes and Silences as Rhetorical Refusal," picks up where the previous chapter left off, in a post-outbreak Minnesota wherein public sector entities were coming together to address Somali autism concerns and vaccine behaviors. This chapter describes one resulting partnership: Midnimo partnered with a human services department to enroll Somali American parents in a microgrant, the Wingham County Autism Grant (WCAG). This chapter first analyzes the documents that made up the WCAG application process. These documents were dynamic sites at which a parent made requests to the state on behalf of a child. This chapter looks closely at the writing practices that the application coordinated or foreclosed and identifies four moments when Somali applicants stopped writing and left the WCAG program. These moments could be read as failures of the grant, signs that Somali applicants needed more guidance, or both, but I read these moments as rhetorical refusals. Accordingly, this chapter follows how and why applicants might deliberately fail to write within institutional documentation as a strategy of outward resistance and inward protection. Rhetorical refusals, enacted at the interface of institutional documentation processes, value the unsupported resources—community, care without surveillance, security, futures that are not geared toward making a child "normal"—that applicants were not willing to give up in exchange for state-sanctioned resources. This chapter then theorizes how rhetorical refusals unfold and signify within one-way, hierarchical, and bureaucratic writing situations and how rhetorical refusals blaze collaborative pathways for rhetoricians as well as policymakers and social service and health professionals to remake institutional processes.

Chapter 4, "The Persuasive Microbiome: Rhetorical Refusal through Care" follows the arcs from participants' refusals to naturopathic, microbiome care. This chapter follows the stories of five Somali American mothers who left the WCAG program and found support under the care of naturopaths who defined autism as an illness resulting from an unbalanced microbiome and prescribed care in the forms of diet, outdoor play, relocation, and other experimental treatments. The chapter begins with an examination of the scientific and popular discourses that describe the microbiome. Microbiome science has introduced a new ontology of the body, one in which the body and its environment are continuous, dynamic, and radically interdependent; at the same time, mainstream microbiome discourses circumscribe this seemingly new body in normative and raced and gendered models of health and illness. Still, mainstream discourses not only act on people but are also acted on by people. Rarely have the ways that marginalized persons use microbiome epistemologies been studied. This chapter explores, through the experience of five Somali American mothers, how these scientific and popular microbiome discourses descended into and were remade within Somali American mothers' healthcare and family relationships, everyday care routines, experiences of community sickness, and heterodox etiologies of autism. This chapter follows how five mothers created daily microbiome-informed domestic practices that also served to translate abstract visions of collective care and community sickness into concrete practices, practices that both provided care for a child and opened new models of care, community, illness, and health. Chapter 4 concludes by identifying five topoi that grounded mothers' microbiome stories and that form a portable rhetorical framework for listening to medical dissent as rhetorical refusal.

CHAPTER 1

Welcome to Health Class

Community Sickness as Rhetorical Refusal's Fertile Ground

There circulates a common explanatory narrative about why Somali families in diaspora suspect their children are part of an unexplained autism cluster. It goes like this: the diagnosis of autism does not exist in Somalia—in fact, there's no equivalent word for autism in the Somali language—and so when Somali children are diagnosed with autism in Western countries, their parents mistakenly, but understandably, conclude that autism must be a Western disease (Decoteau, 2017; Decoteau, 2021). This explanatory narrative is widespread in clinical, public health, social service, and research approaches to understanding Somali autism beliefs. For example, in an interview for this study, one public health official attributed Somali misperceptions about autism to "this notion that since children aren't diagnosed with autism in Somalia that autism, it doesn't exist there. When parents get this diagnosis here, in the US, they think, oh, my child developed this disease here. Maybe, they can get cured if they go back to Africa" (8/15/2018). The University of Minnesota's autism prevalence study, conducted in 2013, also used this explanatory narrative in its opening pages, wherein the authors identified a key concern as the "wide belief [among Somalis] that ASD did not exist in Somalia and that children who have ASD were born abroad" and then traced persisting Somali autism concerns to the possible explanation that "the Somali language lacks words to describe different types of developmental and mental health issues, and this often leads to challenges in communication. For instance, there is no Somali word for autism, and there are only two words to describe the status of individual's mental health ('crazy' and 'sane')" (Hewitt et al., 2013, p. 9). I heard variations of this explanatory narrative many times throughout my fieldwork, from social service staff, public health professionals, healthcare providers, Midnimo staff, and Somali parents. The message was always that Somali persons did not understand autism because they had never encountered the diagnosis and its vocabulary.

A key piece of evidence used to support this explanatory framework was Somalis' nonmedical vocabularies used to refer to illness broadly and autism specifically. Indeed, in my interviews with Somali American parents, parents often referred to autism as "our community's sickness," "our sickness," or "otismo" which translates as "American disease." Sometimes, participants used the terms "community sickness" and "autism" interchangeably to refer to disparate diagnoses. Mothers with children with microcephaly, undiagnosed skin conditions, attention deficit disorder, cerebral palsy, heart conditions, and autism all identified as having children with "our community's sickness." This flexible use of nonmedical language to reference a range of distinct conditions may seem to fit the explanatory narrative that the reason Somali parents do not understand autism is because the diagnosis is unfamiliar. Somali parents' nonmedical, nonspecific autism vocabularies may indeed seem symptomatic of the experience of migrating to a new country with a totally different healthcare system and unfamiliar languages of diagnosis and care. Everything blurs together, and the terms are hard to distinguish. Mistakes happen.

However, I argue in this chapter that Somali parents' alternative vocabularies of autism should not be explained away so easily. The explanation claiming that Somali parents mistake autism for a uniquely Western disease because they have no point of reference for autism is insufficient. This explanation maps onto the literacy frame of approaching dissent in medicine: if only people had better access to medical information, then they would agree with medical guidance. In this chapter, I argue that Somali American parents' persistent use of the term "our community sickness" to describe autism and other illness experiences is not a mistake, is not a translation error, and is not a sign of medical illiteracy. The term *community sickness* is itself a precise term that refers to the social experience of disability, specifically the ways that structural marginalization shapes Somali American families' experiences with autism in nongeneralizable ways. The term *community sickness* defines autism as a social problem, experienced in unique and urgent ways by Somali American families, ways that demand social responses and not necessarily more individualized, medical therapies. For these reasons, Somali American parents used the vocabulary of community sickness, rather than the abstracted, generalizable medical vocabulary of autism. For these reasons, Somali American parents' use of the term *community sickness* and its related discourses of autism (described in this chapter) are a mode of rhetorical refusal, one enacted at the level of language. This mode of rhetorical refusal disengages from medical models of disability and provides protection for families and communities. Here, refusal's exigence is in structural and historical health disparities and systemic inequities, and not in disinformation and translation errors.

This chapter begins in Midnimo's health literacy classroom and describes the content of the health literacy course, which was developed by Midnimo staff to teach Somali American women how to engage American healthcare and how to understand autism as a developmental disability. Somali American students in the course, also mothers of children with autism, scored high on the class quizzes and reported that the health literacy course was valuable. And yet, students also continued to refer to autism as their community sickness. To explore this seeming contradiction, the second half of the chapter turns to Somali students' own definitions of autism, often variations of autism as community sickness. Students invented alternative discourses of autism to describe their own children outside of medical and deficit-based autism etiologies and, often, in line with family genealogies. Parents also devised discourses to explain how dislocation, trauma, ongoing racism, pervasive ableism, and a lack of access to stable housing, safety in public spaces, and fair treatment at school continued to deplete the health of their communities. Parents crafted alternative discourses of autism as community sickness to protect their children and to make public-facing arguments about overlooked social determinants of health. Parents' use of *community sickness* not only depicts a rhetorical refusal in action but also gives voice to the fertile ground (Hausman, 2019) that compelled Somali American parents' medical dissent more broadly, as addressed in the chapters to come.

A New Health Literacy Course: Preparation, Delivery, Evaluation, and Tensions

Malyun, Midnimo's executive director, had envisioned, since the Midnimo's founding, offering a health literacy course taught by Somali women for Somali women. Malyun explained that teaching Somali women about evidence-based medicine and American healthcare was core to Midnimo's mission to empower Somali women. Malyun described health literacy as a critical competency that would empower Somali women with the knowledge to care for their health, to advocate for themselves in clinical encounters, and to recognize if they were getting the care they deserved. Safe and well-planned health literacy classes could bolster Somali women with the confidence and knowledge to seek and benefit from healthcare. In March 2018, Midnimo had received grant funding from a private foundation to offer the center's first health literacy course. The funding was tied to the granting foundation's post-outbreak mission to inform Somali Minnesotans about autism and specified that the health literacy course should focus, in part, on autism and the safety of vaccination. Equipped with funds and parameters, Midnimo staff set out to create their own autism-focused, Somali-centered health literacy curriculum.

The course was created by Sagal and Muna, two program managers at Midnimo, both Somali American women. Sagal had three children, including two sons diagnosed with autism. Sagal had arrived in the US 16 years prior, as a teenager and refugee; she had gone to college in Minnesota and, since graduating, had worked at Minnesota nonprofits. Muna had arrived in the US as a baby with her mother; she had graduated college four years earlier with a degree in public health and, since graduation, had worked at Midnimo. Sagal had resources on hand from having taught health literacy previously; the two program managers used these resources coupled with their own online investigations in health literacy curricula to build Midnimo's curriculum. In addition to the curriculum and in line with the funding requirement that all funded projects develop metrics to quantitatively assess their program's impact, Muna and Sagal created a 15-question pre- and post-test to assess students' learning. Sagal and Muna also created post-course interviews designed to assess whether students planned to change any of their health-related practices based on what they had learned. In the remainder of this section, I describe the course structure and the test results.

Midnimo's Health Literacy Course: Teaching a Medical Discourse of Autism

Midnimo hosted its first health literacy class session in March 2018. Recruitment for the course had been frictionless; most of the organization's staff were Somali American women who lived in close community, and it was never a challenge for Midnimo staff to ask friends, family members, and acquaintances to participate in Midnimo's programming. Twenty women enrolled in the first class, and nineteen completed the course. The health literacy course was ten weeks long; each class spanned 90 minutes and took place on a Monday evening. The class moved along the following schedule, which Sagal and Muna created and outlined in their curriculum materials:

- Class 1: Overall description of health systems (focus: differences between the Somali system and US system)
- Class 2: Preventative care, urgent care, emergency room
- Class 3: Health insurance
- Class 4: Who is who in health services. Types of healthcare and types of providers—examples: pediatric, gynecology, orthodontists, dentist, cardiology, etc.
- Class 5: Pregnancy and childbirth
- Class 6: What to expect at a doctor's office + how to prepare for a visit
- Class 7: ASD: myths + facts; vaccines
- Class 8: ASD: normal development and where/how to seek assessment
- Class 9: ASD: Navigating the resource maze (focus: interpreters, grants, free clinics, mobile health clinics)
- Class 10: Summary

Each class featured a guest speaker, introduced as an expert who worked in healthcare or social services. In a typical class, Sagal and Muna would walk students through a preplanned slide deck in a lecture format. Then, the guest speaker would deliver their own presentation. For the remainder of the class, usually 30 minutes, Sagal and Muna would facilitate discussion.

The first six classes were descriptive and taught students about US healthcare. In the first class, Sagal outlined different kinds of healthcare facilities in the US, including hospitals, outpatient facilities, private clinics, free clinics, community-based clinics, and mobile clinics. Sagal and Muna described different types of providers, such as doctors, nurses, and interpreters. For this lesson, each slide featured a picture of a provider and described how they might be involved in a patient's care. A nurse might take your weight, height, and blood pressure reading; a doctor might come in later for an examination. The goal was to describe the working of US healthcare so that students could understand and use this system. Muna and Sagal localized generic slides to what they knew of their students' concerns. For example, Muna explained the US norms around doctor examinations, and Sagal explained that every patient had the right to an interpreter. She walked students through the steps to request an interpreter and then double-check, before arriving at the clinic, that an interpreter would be present. Each of the classes devoted to US healthcare systems focused heavily on preventative care, which Muna described as an asset of US healthcare and a responsibility of conscientious parents. Sagal spent 20 minutes in one class showing students videos of prenatal classes and telling students that they could take free classes at most hospitals. Muna discussed well-child visits and assured parents that these visits were not designed to find something wrong with their children. Sagal added adamantly that students should not just use preventative medicine for their children. "Tell me this," Sagal told her attentive audience, "what would your family do without you?" (5/16/2018)

The final four courses focused on autism and sought to fit care practices for autistic children into this larger project of mapping American healthcare. The first autism-focused class addressed "myths" about autism. Each slide broadcast a myth, which Muna or Sagal read aloud. They then asked the students to decide if this statement were myth or fact. The first slide read, "Autism doesn't exist in Somalia." Sagal responded, "We all know disability is everywhere." Later, though, Sagal told me that she did think that autism occurred more often and in more severe forms in Somali diaspora children because they had been uprooted from the environment to which their bodies, through generations, had adapted. Still, in the role of teacher, Sagal told her students that autism existed everywhere. She told her students that autism was a genetic condition but that nongenetic and environmental factors might play a role. Sagal elaborated, "All children with autism are different [. . .] but there are symptoms. Does everyone know that word, *symptoms*? It means things that doctors look for to say, yes, that's autism. A cold symptom is a cough." Sagal projected a list of symptoms, which were almost verbatim copied from AutismOne's website and included the following items:

- GI and stomach distress
- delayed speech and language skills
- flat or robotic speech
- echolalia (repeating the same words, sounds, gestures)
- trouble expressing needs and emotions
- trouble relating to others
- repetitive behaviors like hand-flapping, rocking, jumping, or twirling
- constant moving, pacing
- hyper behavior
- fixations on certain activities or objects
- being tied to specific routines
- getting very upset when a routine is disrupted
- extreme sensitivity to touch, light, and sound
- not taking part in imaginary play
- not imitating others' behaviors
- preferring to be alone
- picky eating
- lack of coordination, clumsiness
- impulsiveness (acting without thinking)

- aggressive behavior, both with self and others
- short attention span

Much of this class was spent walking through this list, with parents sharing stories that affirmed and challenged each generalized symptom.

From there, class content shifted to what parents should do to diagnose and support their children. Class 8 featured two visitors, a Somali American program manager named Fadila who worked at an autism therapy center and a white pediatrician named David who worked at a nearby clinic. David walked students through the following developmental milestones and urged parents to contact their pediatrician if a child missed any of them:

- babbling by 12 months
- gesturing by 12 months (waving bye-bye)
- single words by 16 months
- two-word spontaneous phrases by 24-months

David projected a timeline with the ages at which parents should take their children to the pediatrician for well-child visits (3 days old, 2 weeks, 1 month, 2 months, 3 months, 6 months). Well visits, David explained, were the best way to ensure that children were healthy and on track. Next, Fadila explained how to get a child screened for autism. Referring to David's milestones, Fadila said that there were actions a parent could take if a child had missed a milestone or was exhibiting symptoms. Fadila encouraged parents to get an assessment from a licensed psychiatrist or medical doctor, not just from the school, because many health insurance and state services would not accept a school assessment.

The class then focused on therapies for autistic children. Fadila told students that many children, especially children with more severe forms of autism, might benefit from applied behavior analysis (ABA) therapy. Importantly, autistic self-advocates have condemned ABA as an abusive practice because the therapy is focused on "changing the external behaviors of autistic children, with the goal of making an autistic child look and act nonautistic" (Autism Self Advocacy Network, 2022); ABA punishes a person for being themselves and has led to severe negative mental-health outcomes (ASAN, para. 2). But the declamations by autistic people who have been through ABA remain marginalized, and Fadila recommended ABA for autistic children: "What we call ABA, it's an intervention that uses a comprehensive behavioral approach. That means we're addressing everything at once—speech, language, behavior, emotions, rather than having just one person look at each thing. We use positive reinforcement to help children learn appropriate, normal behaviors. It's a great method that doesn't involve all these prescriptions and pills. I know that's a worry for many moms."

Fadila was met with many questions about ABA, and she engaged these questions by speaking experientially about her work; Fadila offered a longer narrative of how ABA might unfold at her center:

> I usually say things like, all of us have triggers. You know when you're going to get upset about something, and you can do something about it. Kids with autism have lots of triggers; we teach them how to notice triggers and respond. We teach them how to control their bodies. We teach them how to relax their bodies. We teach them things like how to transition from one activity to another without getting upset. To teach them about sensory sensitivity, we show them things. We say, see how your child calms down when he holds this? It's because these ridges—here, feel them—calm him down. That's sensory. We teach parents how to make things at home, like slime. A lot of kids love slime. We teach them how to make lava lamps, and, sometimes, if you put toys in rice, kids can really like that, the feeling of the rice.

Fadila's insights into her work compelled much conversation. Follow-up questions turned to the applied, the practical, with students asking about where to find lava lamps and slime and sharing user-generated YouTube instructional videos with one another. Students seemed less interested in the holistic framework of ABA but invested in the specific practices they could mine and make work in their own lives.

David took over the next slide, which asked, "Are there medications for autism?" David offered a succinct response: no. He explained that pharmaceuticals could address some comorbidities that Fadila had mentioned, such as ADHD, insomnia, mood swings, and depression. The next slide moved from pharmaceutical to dietary interventions. David addressed the popular gluten-free, casein-free diet (GF/CF) and explained, "This diet might be helpful to reduce some ASD symptoms or associated behavior problems. The theory behind it is that some children with ASD absorb nutrients differently, and this affects their brain function. But the evidence isn't there. It will cost you a lot of time and money, and there's nothing that says it works."

Many students, however, offered personal stories that diet had produced changes in children's behaviors; students readily offered stories of children who were silent but now participated in school, stories about children who stayed home from school with terrible stomach pains and now played sports. Coursing through the classroom was optimism about the potential of trial-and-error diets. Students asked about how to measure and get more vitamin D to their children, something some had heard could alleviate "autism symptoms." Muna shared that she had heard about a study that suggested that babies who experienced vitamin D deficiency prenatally might develop autism, and so vitamin D supplements might help children "speak more, behave better, not be so hyperactive." Students nodded appreciatively.

David interrupted to clarify: "Yes, some parents say they have noticed a difference in a child's symptoms after starting the GF/CF. But it's all anecdotal—that means just one person's story."

Sagal spoke up in agreement, "Yes, we have learned that there is no medication for autism. Right? There's no medication."

Students mimed agreement to Sagal's statement but continued to swap stories and resources with each other about vitamins and dietary interventions.

•

These scenes account for only slices of the 10-week course, but they provide representative glimpses into how Midnimo's health literacy classes unfolded and how instructors modeled and taught a medical discourse of autism at Midnimo. Across these ten classes, a few themes emerged. The course adhered to a medical definition of autism as an individual debility best treated by medical providers. Even though Sagal and Muna both described to me their own nonmedical views of autism—that autism was caused, in part, by forced migration to an unfamiliar environment and that diet and vitamin regimens could prevent autism, for example—both women, when in the role of teacher, mostly adhered to a medical understanding of autism. In Midnimo's health literacy course, autism was uniformly approached as a pathology with symptoms and unwanted behaviors. The goal was to move a child away from characteristically autistic behaviors and toward an implicit model of a normal child, one that could be mapped along David's milestones. The course deferred to the one-on-one patient-provider consultation as the ultimate source of information and the core site of health decision-making. In these ways, the health literacy course captured one iteration of the medical discourse of autism in action. Participants in the course reported learning from and valuing this medical discourse of autism, but, as the following sections show, this was not the only discourse that parents valued.

Defining Autism: Contradictory Post-Test and Interview Findings

The health literacy course's pre- and post-tests included 15 multiple choice questions designed to assess the extent to which students had learned the health literacy course content and had improved their literacy. The questions about autism included the following:

1. Limited health literacy is associated with:
   A. higher mortality rates
   B. lower levels of health knowledge
   C. greater use of inpatient and emergency department care
   D. poor medicine adherence
   E. B and D
   F. All of the above
   (Correct answer: F)

2. A person with autism can outgrow autism: True or False?
   (Correct answer: False)

3. Autism can be caused by the MMR vaccine: True or False?
   (Correct answer: False)

4. If a child misses one of these milestones, you should make a doctor's appointment for the child. Check all milestones that apply:
   A. Babbling by 12 months
   B. Responding to their name by nine months
   C. Smiling back at you by nine months
   D. Pointing by nine months
   E. Can follow instructions by two years old
   F. Can read by two years old
   (Correct answers: A, B, C, D, E)

5. List three common symptoms of autism:
   (Correct answers include, for example, robotic speech, echolalia, trouble expressing needs, trouble relating to others, repetitive behaviors, pacing, and more)

6. Underline three services that insurance will cover for a child diagnosed with autism:
   (Correct answers from a list are as follows: applied behavioral analysis [ABA], speech therapy, a personal care assistant [PCA] [can be a family member])

Students performed better on their post-tests than on their pre-tests, and this metric suggested that students had learned about medicine, autism, and health systems in the course. In other words, students had improved their health literacy. The primary outcome of the course had been met. But the interviews designed to elicit students' health beliefs and predicted health behaviors told a different story. These interviews consisted of four semistructured questions designed to learn what students planned to do with the information they had gained from the course. First, students were asked if they felt they had learned valuable things. Of the 18 students who participated in interviews, all 18 reported that they had learned valuable information. All 18 students reported that they were happy they took this course. Seventeen students stated that, given the chance to go back in time, they would participate in the course again.

The second question asked students about any changes they planned to make on account of what they had learned in the course. Ten participants reported that there were things they planned to do differently. Three participants said that they planned to pursue an autism screening for a child. One participant reported that she would go to urgent care rather than the emergency room. One participant planned to take her family to the dentist, and one participant planned to get a mammogram. Four participants had plans to pursue services at Fadila's clinic. As well, eight students reported that they did not plan to make any changes. When students didn't offer up a possible change, Sagal or Muna would ask if they had feedback, anything that would make the course more relevant to them, perhaps. No one offered any concrete suggestions. For example, when Muna interviewed Farah, who reported that she had liked the class but had not learned anything that would change her health-related routines, the conversation unfolded as follows:

MUNA: Is there anything you think would be useful for other mothers to have?
FARAH: No. We're used to it, to—how to deal.
MUNA: But is there anything that would help?
FARAH: Advice, I love it. Yes, yes, I love advice.
MUNA: And is there advice you wished you had gotten in this class? Like, around a certain topic?
FARAH: No. This class was very good. (8/20/2018)

Farah's response is representative of the responses of the eight participants who reported that they could not think of any changes they planned to make. These participants reported that they had enjoyed the course, did not have any critical feedback, *and* they had no planned changes to report.

The third question asked students how they would define autism now that they had completed the course. All students had ready definitions, and none of their definitions could be mapped onto the medical definition of autism advanced in the health literacy course. The following list includes all definitions offered by the 18 mothers who completed the course and participated in a post-course interview. I include these definitions in full because they express how a diverse group of students all advanced definitions of autism as community sickness that could not be separated from their experiences of dislocation, home loss, diaspora, and structural precarity. Participants' definitions are as follows:

- Autism is something that will be with us for our lives. It is how my son sees the world. It means he struggles with his emotions. It means that as his mother, I need to help. If there's one thing I need to teach him, it's to recognize when a feeling is coming up and do something about it. Because right now he is small, but what happens when he's a teenager? This is my mission as a mother. What happens if he has that rage as a teenager? I won't be able to control him.
- It's genetic. Neurological. It's something they study. But I see my son as a blessing. I see my son as a blessing, and I need to care for him. Sometimes he runs away because he's in his own head. It's just, I can't describe it, but he goes somewhere else, his brain goes into its own world, and he can get lost. Every time he comes back, I could yell at him, but I hug him. I rub his back.
- It's a sickness. It's affecting our children. It takes away their voices, their stories.
- Autism is a sickness that is taking away our children. We are a nation of poets, and our children can't speak. They hide under tables and run away. My son can't put two words together. My father was a poet. It's a sickness that is hurting our children in Minnesota, in Ohio, in Canada.
- I say, like Rain Man, and then everyone knows. There is more stigma for our children. It's different for our children. They don't speak, they have more stomach distress. They suffer more.
- Kids that are delayed. Speech delay, social delay, learning delay, they cannot talk, they cannot communicate with other children. For my child, he doesn't speak. When my child was one year old, we noticed that my child was not talking. I told the doctor that my child wasn't talking, and I needed to know why. My child's doctor said my child has a speech delay, he would grow out of it, every child is different, but I already knew that my child has autism. And it turned out that my child has autism. Even the doctors don't know what it is. None of them know why our community has the most autism, and never mild autism.
- It's a sickness. Autism is a sickness.

- Autism is a sickness. You can't define it. You know Tom Cruise? Tom Cruise has autism. So does Assad [my son]. For Assad, it is mostly he repeats things and gets upset if things are out of order. If I say, We're late, then the whole car ride, he'll say, We're late, we're late, we're late. If we take back roads, he gets very upset. I just take the same route because it calms him. But he's so sweet, he's so compassionate, he hugs so much. The teachers love him. Everyone can see a sweet kid, and everyone loves a sweet kid. He has Asperger's, so you really must pay attention.
- It's a sickness of the mental kind. It's stigmatized in our community because people don't understand.
- It's a sickness. I believe it is from vitamin D deficiency and from lack of sun and layers of clothes.
- Autism means you have a unique mind. No one wanted me to get my son diagnosed. There are uncles, grandfathers, others who are quiet and different. But I think a diagnosis would help him; he's very smart. With autism, there are things that are different, and sometimes children can't speak, which is hard. But you have to listen and give them love, and you'll learn how they think and feel. My son is very introverted, he doesn't speak.
- Autism, there isn't a cure; it's a spectrum. It's different for every child, that's why they call it a spectrum. Our children don't have language. Our children never have the Asperger's form.
- My son developed a bad case of stuttering after he received the vaccine. He went from having a clear speech to not being able to say two sentences without stuttering. His doctor said it was a coincidence. I can understand why the parents are afraid to give their kids live vaccinations like the measles. I wish someone would do a study of it in Somalia. If it's higher there, then it means that it's genetic. If it's higher here, maybe it's the vaccines or the food.
- In our community, autism can be a taboo topic. Anything related to mental health, to autism is taboo. It's our community sickness. And the more we talk about it, then there's nothing to be ashamed about. Our children are our blessings, and we love them. We also are the only ones who know how it's hurting our children. Is it the vaccines? The food? The climate? We need to talk to each other and put one and one together.
- It's a sickness; autism is worse for Somali children. White children have the less severe versions, Asperger's. Somali children are very delayed, many don't speak. The reality is autism is seen as very negative.
- Autism is a sickness hurting our community. Our children cannot speak. We don't know how it is caused. Is it the vaccines? From foods? Because we live in toxic places? Is it because we aren't meant for winter?

- Autism is a developmental delay. It's a mental disability. It's worse for Somalis. People with autism look normal, but they might not speak, or they might not be able to communicate like others. Maybe they scream for no reason. Maybe they're quiet. I have not come across a child that looks so normal as my son, but he is different. That makes it hard because people see your son hitting or screaming and they think, what's wrong with you? Why did you raise your child like that? Some people think children grow out of autism, that it's a bad idea to diagnose them. But I don't believe that, and I'm not ashamed of autism.
- Autism . . . I can't tell you. It is our community's sickness. But I can tell you about my daughter. She is very creative. She loves to draw. She plays on the iPad, she loves computer games. She doesn't speak. She has a lot of joy. There's a reason they call autism a spectrum. It is different for everyone.

These definitions show that even as students learned, appreciated, and demonstrated mastery of the health literacy course's content, students held firm to their own definitions of autism, the very definitions that the health literacy course was designed to correct and replace. What value did these unsanctioned definitions hold? Why did participants maintain that autism was a community sickness? The next section engages these questions by identifying five protective and participatory discourses that unfurled from these definitions.

Five Discourses of Autism as Community Sickness

Across health literacy students' definitions of autism were threaded five discourses of autism as community sickness, which I describe in this section. In the first discourse, a protective one, participating mothers genealogized autism and crafted personal definitions of autism, each unique to a specific child and their lineage. Second, participants depicted a social model of disability, one that called for social change rather than individual therapies. Third and relatedly, some students used *autism* to reference a specific social model of disability, one that insisted on autism as a distinct experience for Somali refugees. Fourth, participants used *autism* as an affiliative code word, one that signaled a shared experience of autism in Somali diaspora and a shared understanding of community sickness; this affiliative discourse was useful to build biosocial coalitions, bounded by shared social experiences of illness and aimed at change. Fifth, participants used *autism* to refer to a physiologically different diagnosis for Somalis; this aberrant discourse demonstrates how participants drew on their own embodied experiences to contest science—and to continue to contest science even as they were repeatedly told their concerns were wrong, were symptoms of wrong thinking. These discourses of autism speak to the fertile ground that seeded Somali participants' rhetorical refusals in this and other contexts.

Discourse 1: Autism as Genealogized Difference

When asked to define autism, ten students did so by describing their own children—their personalities, stories, idiosyncrasies, and the singular experience of parenting them. These students created discursive space to describe their children on their own terms and not in accordance with a diagnostic profile. One student defined autism as "how my son sees the world." Another mother explained, "I've learned about autism through my son. I see my son as a blessing. He teaches me." In a similar reorientation, Sahra declined to offer a universalizing definition for autism and instead spoke about her irreducible daughter: "Autism . . . I can't tell you. But I can tell you about my daughter. She is very creative. She loves to draw. She plays on the I-pad, she loves computer games. She doesn't speak" (8/30/2018). Sahra did not distinguish between more categorically autistic traits ("she doesn't speak") and more socially normal traits ("she is very creative"). Sahra simply described her daughter as a multifaceted person. In doing so, Sahra redefined autism from a medical disability and made rhetorical space to "welcome a child on grounds other than biomedical normalcy" (Rapp, 1999, p. 190). In place of standard definitions, students crafted anecdotes, character sketches, and stories about their children. Parents refused a standardized, deficit-based medical definition accompanied by a list of general symptoms. Parents redefined autism in line with their own, indelible children, as individuals with their own traits, desires, pasts, and unfolding futures.

Some parents defined autism in a way that connected their children to family lineages. Amina defined autism by describing her son and then explaining that her son had a distinct mind like his other family members: "Autism means you have a unique mind. No one wanted me to take my son to get diagnosed. There are uncles, grandfathers, others who are quiet and different." In a later interview, Sofia also wove her son's possible autism into her family lineage and explained that her son's lack of speech was an inheritance of his grandfather's and uncle's quiet demeanors—a family trait to be treasured, not diagnosed and corrected. Sofia referred to her son and his uncle and grandfather as "late bloomers." While the health literacy curriculum pathologized autism, these mothers genealogized autism (Rapp, 1999, p. 175). Through familial discourses, participants reclaimed autism by de-medicalizing and destigmatizing autism and then recontextualizing *autism* as a term useful to describe their children and to embed their children in genealogies of esteemed family members. Participants used the term to weave together sundered family trees and to recognize traits passed down through generations. In return, the word *autism* made a bubble of privacy around a family, a space where autism could be made their own, defined in their own terms, in accordance with a specific child, and in reverence to kin—all without outside medical and state incursions and corrections.

Discourse 2: Autism as a Socially Constructed Problem

The next two discourses of autism take activist, outward-facing approaches. In this second discourse, participants used the word *autism* to advance a social model of disability. When asked to define autism, five students described autism as a condition shaped by external biases. Ashwaq first defined autism in general and deficit-based terms, while also emphasizing that autism more severely affected Somali American families: "Autism is a developmental delay. It's a mental disability. It's worse for Somalis. People with autism look normal, but they might not speak, or they might not be able to communicate like others" (8/30/2018). Then, Ashwaq explained that autism was hard because of the uninformed judgment a family could attract: "I have not come across a child that looks so normal as my son, but he is different. That makes it hard because people see your son hitting or screaming, and they think, what's wrong with you? Why did you raise your child like that?" Ashwaq concluded her definition with the firm statement that "I am not ashamed of autism." Ashwaq ended her definition with a reaffirmation that autism itself is not shameful, but people and structures, the outside world, make autism hard.

Four other students defined autism by the stigma attached to it. One student offered as a definition that "it's a sickness of the mental kind. It's stigmatized in our community because people don't understand" (8/29/2018). Another student defined autism as follows: "In our community, autism can be a taboo topic. Anything related to mental health, to autism is taboo. But it's also our community sickness. And the more we talk about it, then there's nothing to be ashamed about. Our children are our blessings, and we love them" (9/3/2018). One mother, Suad, who had defined autism as "a sickness of the mental kind," then offered a story about the social construction of disability:

> The thing is that the taboo issue, disability, is also what's preventing them [Somali parents] from using one another, because they are used to things like, you know, they say, "Oh, that kid's crazy," the judgment, and that kind of thing. My older brother has polio, and I remember all the nasty things that people would say to him, so it is a taboo, and it's another page that we need to open these days, a community conversation saying how we treat people with disability. (8/30/2018)

Suad repeatedly identified the problem as stigma, not as autism. After my interview with Suad, a community health worker, who had been helping with translation, turned to me, and said that she could relate to a lot of these interviews, especially in their focus on experiences of external judgment. She explained,

> When I go to teach classes or speak at places, people say, there's that infertile woman or the woman who can't have kids. They don't even mean it in a rude way, but that doesn't mean, when I go home at night, it doesn't hurt. I'm very strong, but when I go home at night, it hurts. It's not a rude thing, but it's a bad culture. We say, it's ok, but, no, it really hurts. They say it's not a problem, but it is a problem. It hurts, and we need to have ways to prevent that hurt. (8/28/2018)

"A bad culture"—it was a way of capturing a social model of disability. These participants' responses were invested in naming stigma and changing social norms that stigmatized autism.

Although the discussions in the health literacy courses kept coming back to the question of how to eliminate autism symptoms, students' own definitions of autism suggest that few participants saw autism as an inherent problem. Students saw the world that judged and hemmed in their autistic children as a problem. Accordingly, when students were asked to define autism, students rarely focused on the medical definitions and symptom lists that they had spent the last few months learning. Students used autism as a jumping-off point to carefully describe their own children, to address the problem of stigma, and to imagine different worlds where the social norms that made certain forms of difference disabling were remade. These definitions of autism advocate for a social model of disability, one in which disability is not a medical problem, rooted in deficiencies in individual bodies, but a social problem, one upheld by alterable structural conditions that exclude full participation in society (Kerschbaum, 2014; Hamraie, 2017; Konrad, 2018).

Further illustrative of this understanding of autism as a social problem, Kamal, a Somali American owner of a PCA agency, told me about a father he had helped:

> One family I know, an autistic nine-year-old girl. She got out [of their house], and she ran through the streets. And she was dancing in the streets. Dancing, just dancing. And then, someone called the police. And I guess the police were around, and they came and took up the girl, and they took her to her house. They knocked on the door, and the dad answered, and they said, "Do you know where your daughter was?" And he said, "Last I saw her, we were both sleeping." And they said, "She was dancing in the street." You know what the father did? He took her back to a village in Somalia where there are no cars. (5/20/2018)

Kamal's retelling of his friend's experience suggests that the dancing girl's father did not vie to change his daughter's personality or behaviors. This father sought to find an environment where his daughter would be safe to dance in the streets. Often, when I spoke with medical professionals, they would express frustration with Somali American parents who wanted to care for their children with autism through reverse migration to Somalia. Many healthcare professionals understood this inclination as grounded in the erroneous belief that autism was a Western disease. However, Kamal's story suggests an alternative motivation for reverse migration—not the hope that a child would be "cured" of autism, but the hope that a child would enjoy an environment wherein they were less surveilled and stigmatized. Importantly, this vision of return migration as a portal to a better life was not universal, and many participants explained that disability was stigmatized in Somalia. But the point here is not to compare what cultures are more and less ableist; whether this father's hope for a more accommodating life in Somalia was warranted, his story suggests that some parents desired not to change their children but to find a place where their children could thrive. Accordingly, students used this second discourse to advance a social model of disability, one in which autism is a community sickness because of stigma and structural exclusion.

Discourse 3: Autism as a Social Problem Shaped by Racialization

In a third and related discourse, nine students advanced a more specific social model of disability, one that spoke to how autism was disabling to Somali people in Minnesota in nongeneralizable ways. When asked to define autism, nine students answered that autism was a community sickness unique to Somali families in Western diaspora. One mother offered the following definition: "It's a sickness. It's affecting our children. It takes away their voices, their stories"

(8/30/2018). Another mother described autism as "a sickness that is taking away our children. We are a nation of poets, and our children here can't speak" (8/29/2018). In these Somali-specific definitions, participants refused to assimilate their distinct autism experiences into a one-size-fits-all medical definition. Instead, Somali American participants defined autism in ways that insisted that their experiences of home loss and forced migration as well as structural precarity and racism in resettlement shaped their experience of autism.

Specifically, students' definitions of autism incorporated experiences of racism and surveillance at school, public perceptions of Black boys and men as threatening, and gendered stereotypes about Somali mothers. To this first point, parents frequently described intensified disciplining of their children at school. Asha said that when her son expressed verbal anger at the bullying he endured at school, the school responded by having administrators search him every day for weapons (1/10/2018). Anab attributed the autism-related challenges her family faced to the ways that peers and school officials perceived her son as a threat:

> He doesn't have friends. He was bullied a lot at camp. And [at school] they search his backpack now, to make sure he doesn't have weapons, and he hates that. No one talks to him about it, they just do it. I want people to understand that he has a disease and to help him understand his disease. I want people to tell him, you have a disease, but you can still study, you can still do well, this disease does not mean that you can't study. I want people to make him love school. (2/1/2018)

Stories like Asha's and Anab's align with a large body of scholarship documenting racial disparities in school discipline and showing that, in the US, Black students are disproportionately represented in school discipline settings (Skiba et al., 2002; US Department of Education Office for Civil Rights, 2014; Nowicki, 2018). Such experiences were intensified for Somali American boys in post-9/11 Minnesota, where Somali youth faced suspicion that they were interacting with terrorist groups and resultant surveillance and over-policing (Abdi, 2015a). Nasra described the preventative steps she took to advocate for her second-grade son and to preempt teachers and administrators from regarding her son as unintelligent, disrespectful, or threatening; Nasra described her vigilance:

> I don't give them any reason to think he's bad or unintelligent—I have to be ahead on everything. At school, I come, I hug the principal. I am always there to drop them off. I meet the teachers once a week. If I am meeting the

teachers, I make sure to get eight hours of sleep. I want to be ready to go. And I have to be. You have to be on top of everything, meeting the teachers, going to the morning breakfasts, I never miss anything.

Nasra reported feeling positive about the improvements her son was making at school, but her description shows the heaps of preparation, rhetorical labor, and emotional energy that she devoted to advocating for her son and making sure that school personnel saw him as a boy trying to learn and not as a lost cause. To talk about autism, for these participants, was to talk about discrimination, bias, and surveillance.

Participants also spoke to their fears that their sons would be perceived as threats as they grew into teenagers and men. Farax, a health literacy student, defined autism in the following terms:

> Autism is something that will be with us for our lives. It is how my son sees the world. It means he struggles with his emotions. It means that as his mother, I need to help. If there's one thing I need to teach him, it's to recognize when a feeling is coming up and do something about it. Now he is small, but what happens when he's a teenager? This is my mission as a mother. What happens if he has that rage as a teenager? I won't be able to control him. (9/1/2018)

Farax dealt with autism in an outside world that viewed Black men with fear and reacted with violence. In her definition of autism, Farax could not—or would not—abstract the medical diagnosis from her social experience of raising a Somali American boy in a racist, violent world. In these stories, parents didn't just navigate a world that stigmatized disability; parents contended with specific threats that materialized at the intersections of racist and ableist surveillance and policing structures.

This third discourse demonstrates how Somali American parents' shared definition of autism as community sickness was a synecdoche for what rhetorician Suban Cooley Nur (2023) has called the assemblage of "becoming Black" in the African diaspora. Nur positions the term "becoming Black" as distinct from "being Black" and as useful to name the ways that "Black bodies are racialized in a Western context" (p. 258). Nur describes being Black as connected with the "largeness and vastness of Black aliveness" and describes in more detail how

> the vitality of Black aliveness thrives and grows beyond the challenges of violent displacements and ruptures of culture, carried across borders as

language, music, food, art, story, and more, transforming and living on in new geographic locations as displaced peoples carve, weave, blend, and rebuild elements of a culture for those who can no longer experience it as it was. (p. 262)

To "become Black," on the other hand,

is a determinant of the world experiencing you in your Blackness; it is how you are perceived in the non-Black world, treated by non-Black people, and how Black people between themselves also manifest a mistreatment of one another through a hierarchy of systemic situations imposed on intersecting Black identities (you know . . . whiteness). (p. 263)

Participants built into their definitions an argument that the forced experience of "becoming Black" in the US cannot be extricated from Somali American families' experiences with autism. To define autism as an abstract, medical entity is to define autism in terms of the dominant, white experience, is to void Somali American families' experiences and most urgent concerns. Thus, students continued to define autism through a social model of disability that focused on how structural racism made autism a specific experience for Somali families in Minnesota.

In a final example of how racist structures shaped Somali parents' experiences of autism, Midnimo hosted two parent advocates at a workshop for Somali parents with children with autism. One speaker, Hodo, was a Somali American woman, a mother of four children, including two with autism, and a parent liaison in the public schools. The second speaker, Laurel, was a white woman, a mother of two children with autism, and a speaker and consultant about autism and parenting. Laurel opened the workshop by introducing herself and telling her story. She told the assembled Somali parents about her own children with autism and her role as a single mother. She focused on how she came to be an advocate for other parents. She explained that her goal was to empower mothers and to foster a support group atmosphere, one wherein all participants could "open our hearts" to one another (8/25/2018). The first thing Laurel offered the mothers in attendance was a set of business-sized cards that read "Please be kind, my child has autism" on one side, and, on the reverse side, read "For more information or to offer your support: Autism Society of MN: www.ausm.org." Laurel explained that she gave these cards to people in public places, like the library or a playground, to preempt others from judging her and being rude to her children. She explained, "These cards can help. I've had experiences where people are rude to me. Where they might stare at my children, say something under their breath, comment loudly that the library is for reading, you all know what I mean. After I've handed my cards—I don't say anything, just hand a card and walk away—they've come up to me, they've apologized, and they've thanked me for giving them the chance to learn and rethink their initial responses."

Hodo, the second guest speaker, interjected, "I don't know if we are ready for these cards. We go to the library, and our child acts up, and people don't just see a child having a tantrum. They see a woman in a hijab, someone who is not like them. They see a woman with six kids and think, why did you have so many kids if you can't control them? They see a woman who doesn't know English, and they think you're dumb. No one helps. They all stare. I love the library, the mall, the parks, but it is too much work for us to go there."

Mothers in attendance nodded in agreement.

Malyun said, "Racism."

Malyun's one-word summary—racism—is an appropriate one with which to end this section. It is the reason that parents' use of community sickness to speak about autism was accurate, incisive. Autism was not the same for Laurel as it was for Hodo. Autism, as a medical diagnosis, was not useful to express these differences, to voice the stress-inducing, relentless intersections of racialization, otherization, and disability. By refusing to have their own racialized experiences of autism absorbed into a medical definition, parents also refused to stop talking about the ways that racist structures hurt their children.

Discourse 4: Autism as an Affiliative Codeword

Somali parents used this fourth, affiliative discourse of community sickness, first, to voice the ways that social structures and deep inequities made autism a specific challenge for Somali families in the US, and then to find each other, to support each other, and to share resources. The following story of Nur's speech exemplifies how Somali American parents used autism and community sickness as in-group code words to gather Somali parents around shared experiences and to circulate situational advice. After the health literacy class, Sagal told me that I couldn't write about autism without hearing Nur. Nur belonged to a category that had proven elusive in my fieldwork, Somali fathers of children with autism. Sagal told me that everyone knew Nur: "He started off by speaking all over, neighborhood meetings, political things, the mall—I'm serious, wherever he could speak, he would" (8/4/2018). Now, Sagal explained, his presence was requested. She told me Nur could often be found advocating for more autism resources for Somali families at the Capitol but that he always returned to his community and often gave speeches at mosques and malls. At the talk I attended, Nur addressed the crowd in Somali, and Sagal translated along for me:

> He's saying, I want to tell you all two things about me. I have two sons with autism. I've been evicted from my apartment 17 times. Seventeen times! We can afford rent, but with 17 evictions, no one wants to rent to us. My sons—if you have autism, you know it—but my sons will destroy the furniture, the walls, the floors. They'll make a lot of noise. Every time we rent a place, we get kicked out. My family has been homeless many times. What I want to tell you is: autism will get you evicted. It will leave you homeless. You must do whatever you can to not have autism. I don't want anyone else to have to deal with this—17 evictions, no home. Protect your children, do not let them get autism. That's why I'm here to tell you: you cannot let your baby get the MMR vaccine. I'm telling you, if your child gets autism, it's evictions, it's homelessness, it's impossible. (9/5/2018)

At first, I was surprised and, I admit, disappointed. I had hoped for a new angle from Nur and had not expected an antivaccination speech. Yet, as I listened, I noticed that Nur did not spend time laying out any evidence that the MMR vaccine caused autism. Rather, he spoke about his evictions and housing instability. He spoke about his sons' expensive and set-in-their-ways therapists, about copays and transportation. He said that his sons did learn from their therapists, which was more than he could say about what his sons gleaned from school. "They're always suspended," he told the crowd. "They spend their days in a room with a para, doing nothing, getting angry, hating school. If you have a child with autism, there isn't a school for them."

Nur described autism wholly as a social problem that manifested in specific ways for Somali people in the US—in evictions, discrimination, children left behind at school, and parents overtaxed and without support. Here, autism was community sickness, a set of interlocking risks and harms caused by social inequality and locked in place by systemic racism and ableism. Nur's speech engages the second and third discourses of autism as community sickness, but Nur's words also branch into a new discourse, a strategic one used by and for Somalis in diaspora. In Nur's speech, *autism*, the word, was useful for signaling to Somali parents who had similar experiences. When Nur used *autism* to refer not to a medical diagnosis but to community sickness, to talk about evictions and community protection and vaccines, then other Somali parents knew what he was talking about, knew that he had been through what they had been through, and they listened.

Nur explained to parents how to survive not autism but community sickness, that is, the experience of disability as a Somali person in a structurally inequitable, hostile Western world. Nur's use of *autism* as an affiliative code word helped illuminate the ways that other parents, mentioned throughout this study, had been sharing with each other adaptive tactics geared toward surviving the structural conditions that shaped the experience of parenting a Somali child with autism in the US. In the health literacy course, parents traded experiential anecdotes about what had worked for them—diets, therapist referrals, vitamin routines. In these exchanges, *autism* functioned as an in-group signal, a word that, if you knew what to listen for, could gesture to the Somali diaspora experience of autism without having to unpack the trauma of home loss, war, migration, resettlement, racism, and precarity. From there, parents could exchange heterodox, localized strategies that derived from and responded to their own, nongeneralizable experiences of autism. These constrained, on-the-ground strategies were geared toward protecting their families right now, right here, with whatever scant resources were on hand. If that included nonvaccination, so be it; greater threats loomed.

Discourse 5: Somali Autism Clusters as Real

Across students' definitions of autism, there was also threaded another, different discourse. This fifth discourse does not necessarily advance a social model of disability. This discourse does not necessarily inform the argument that autism is a distinct experience for Somalis in diaspora because of structural marginalization and the intensified ways that ableism, racism, anti-Muslim discrimination and hate, and xenophobia intersect in their day-to-day lives. Rather, some students described autism as a distinct experience for their Somali children because autism was physiologically different for Somali children in diaspora than it was for non-Somali children. In the 18 definitions participants advanced about autism, nine participants stated plainly that autism was physiologically different for Somali children. These parents defined autism as, in one participant's definition, "a sickness that is taking away our children" (8/29/2018). Participants built their definitions around the claim that autism was different for them, and not just for social or structural reasons. One participant specified, "It's different for our children. They don't speak, they have more stomach distress. They suffer more." Another participant defined autism by claiming, "It's worse for Somalis." Three participants specified that Somali children experienced more severe forms of autism. Three parents, in their definitions, offered potential reasons for their beliefs that autism was a different physiological condition for Somali children; these parents posited that vaccinations, climate, lack of sun and vitamin D, food sources, and abrupt changes and displacements could be sources of a new, poorly understood kind of autism manifesting in a cluster among Somali children in the Western diaspora.

This fifth discourse is the one most easily dismissed as wrong, for the reason that its adherents need more scientific and medical education. But in the chapters to come, I argue that arguments such as this one can be read as rhetorical refusals with potential epistemic value. This argument is a harder one to make. Indeed, many humanists and social scientists are more comfortable advancing arguments about the social implications of nonscientific action or the structural reasons that trust in expertise breaks down. I, too, am more inclined to look at the ways that acts of medical dissent—wrong uses of autism, nonvaccination, investment in wellness trends—might be idioms for larger issues, might be rejections less against science than against medical racism, medical models of disability, or the interplay of profit, politics, and pharmaceuticals. It's harder to take seriously claims that are nonscientific, such as "the MMR vaccine can cause autism," "Somali children do not have Asperger's," or "autism only occurs in the global North." But when it comes to taking participants and interlocutors seriously, then it's also important to take seriously these sorts of claims.

In doing so, we might see Somali American parents' suspicions and nonmedical convictions as the beginning of a citizen science–aligned movement. In this frame, it does not sound so antiscience to consider that a group of marginalized individuals might advance a real health concern, dismissed by the experts but undeniable in their own embodied experiences. Indeed, many citizen science movements began with a few nonspecialists who insisted that their embodied knowledge and lived expertise *were real,* even though experts said otherwise. Such movements have led to medical advancement and knowledge building, in cases as far-ranging as AIDS/HIV (Epstein, 1996), environmentally caused cancer clusters (Brown, 2007; McCormick et al., 2004), PFAS contamination (Ohayon et al., 2023), radiation poisoning (Kimura, 2016), reproductive healthcare and prescription birth-control (Kline, 2010), multiple chemical sensitivity (Alaimo, 2010), and long COVID (Ireson et al., 2022). Too, many pharmaceutical products have been recalled or amended with a black box when they proved dangerous to certain populations, often delimited on racial and ethnic lines (Fejerman et al., 2014; Bichell, 2015; Oh et al., 2015; Vogel, 2015; Shukla et al., 2021). Sociologists Harry Collins and Robert Evans (2002) have coined the term "contributory expertise" to argue that lay knowledge or beliefs, when they contradict scientific consensus or knowledge, do not have to be instantly dismissed as wrong or as antiscience; instead, these beliefs might be seen as the grounds for future scientific study, as the seeds of new research questions to explore.

I explore these cases and arguments further in chapter 2, wherein I ask the question, What if the risks that Somali American participants posit about vaccines are real? Or, at least, What if we listen to these risks as real? In chapter 2, I advance the argument that rhetorical refusals can have epistemic value, can productively contest science, and can advance scientific and medical knowledge. But, to close this section, it is important to also listen to participants' autism definitions as making claims about the physiological nature of autism. These definitions demonstrate that students did not trust that general medical knowledge applied to them. Students felt that their somatic experiences were outside of the purview of medicine. As one student imagined in her definition of autism, "I wish someone would do a study of [autism] in Somalia. If it's higher there, then it means that it's genetic. If it's higher here, maybe it's the vaccines or the food." This student was not against science, but she did believe that science had not caught up to her embodied experiences as a refugee in the US. Fellow students felt that their embodied experiences of warfare, famine, displacement, and forced migration marked their bodies in ways that made medical knowledge nonapplicable to them. Were these claims accurate? That question is outside of the scope of my study and expertise, but, as I argue in the chapters to come, listening to—rather than trying to educate away or trying to explain away—these embodied convictions could make for better medicine. That is, medical dissent and refusal can, sometimes, flag real yet unstudied health problems and can contribute to new scientific knowledge.

•

Together, these interwoven discourses of autism as community sickness tell a polyvocal counterstory to the widely circulating stock story that Somali parents calling autism a Western disease, or a community sickness, or otismo was wrong and a symptom of lacking health literacy (Martinez, 2020). In each of these incorrect uses of *autism* and *community sickness*, Somali American parents, yes, defined autism in nonmedical and scientifically incorrect terms but also argued that their own experiences of autism were shaped by their histories of displacement and loss and their present, daily experiences of structural exclusion, precarity, and marginalization. It was these experiences that parents referred to when they used the term *community sickness*. It was the lived experience of community sickness that formed the fertile ground of parents' refusals to adopt a medical approach to autism, an argument I take up in the next two sections.

Rhetorical Refusal through Wrong Discourses

In the post-test evaluations required by Midnimo's health literacy course's funders, any student's expression of autism as community sickness was coded as wrong. These misuses of *autism* and *community sickness* were explained as symptoms of poor health literacy and were positioned as addressable with better health education. Sociologist Clare L. Decoteau (2021), however, has pointed out that "there is an implicit colonialist presumption that Somalis' hesitation around accepting a particular categorical description of autism signifies a 'backward' approach to mental illness" (p. 42). Health literacy frameworks "presume that people who do not accept Western categories and therapeutics have no means of explaining or healing psychological distress" (p. 44). The explanatory narrative that Somalis do not understand autism because there is no similar diagnosis in the Somali language relies on this presumption. Somali students' discourses of community sickness, described above, challenge this explanatory narrative and demonstrate that Somali students' expressions of community sickness are not "backward" approaches to illness and are not signs of an absence of "means of explaining or healing psychological distress" (p. 42).

The opposite, these five discourses are precise ways to speak about the lived experience of autism in Somali diaspora. Somali students' uses of alternative and wrong discourses about autism were rhetorical refusals, that is, communicative acts of dissent against medical ways of knowing and caring for autism. As rhetorical refusals, these alternative discourses do provide "means of explaining or healing psychological distress" (Decoteau, 2021, p. 44). Participants' rhetorical refusals "explain" autism through a social model of disability that explains how systemic racism and ableism as well as the daily lived experience of structural precarity define autism for Somalis in Minnesota. These intentional discourses, as rhetorical refusals, make visible the social, structural, and ideological conditions that stigmatize certain populations and disabilities and position certain populations as structurally vulnerable to health risks. Participants' rhetorical refusals also proffer tactics to "heal" this experience of autism through collective care networks and heterodox strategies, including microbiome care, as described in chapter 4, that respond not to neurobiological symptoms of autism but to the lived experience of autism for Somalis in the US.

Referring to autism as "our community's sickness," Somali American students rerouted attention away from the neurological, biological mechanisms of autism and toward the social norms that construct autism as a disability in particular ways for Somalis in diaspora. Medical anthropologist Christina Zarowsky's work on post-traumatic stress disorder (PTSD) among Somalis in Ethiopia (2000) has shown that Somalis rejected PTSD for similar and instructive reasons; the diagnosis PTSD rendered an individual malady what many participants described as a collective political injury, one wrought by external, geopolitical events, including war, famine, and forced migration. Participating Somalis regarded their mental distress as a shared response to warfare, dispossession, and the threat of annihilation; this distress was a starting place for deserved anger and political action (p. 398). PTSD, by contrast, was a clinical category that prescribed individualized, pharmaceutical treatments and thereby "bracketed power, history, culture, and politics" (p. 400). Participating Somalis rejected PTSD not because they did not understand or were shamed by the diagnosis but because they rejected the ways PTSD was abstracted from politics and addressed in a private, one-on-one therapeutic relationship that stymied collective anger and action.

Similarly, Somali students in Midnimo's health literacy class used the discourses of community sickness to reject the health literacy course's depoliticization of their experiences of autism. Mainstream medical explanations, like those taught in the health literacy course, "naturalize and individualize a condition that is lived very differently by populations, depending on their social locations" (Decoteau, 2021, p. 216). This is because "science has a tendency to ignore the fact that cultural, structural, and ideological conditions have also carved up the world, rendering particular populations vulnerable to poor health conditions, lower life expectancies, and higher levels of distrust and discrimination" (Decoteau, 2021, p. 216). Somali participants' use of *autism* as "community sickness" reintegrated autism into the "cultural, structural, and ideological conditions" (Decoteau, 2021, p. 216) and unbracketed "power, history, culture, and politics" (Zarowsky, 2000, p. 400) that shaped students' lived experiences of autism.

And so, after completing the health literacy course, Somali American students continued to use *autism* to refer to community sickness for intentional, rhetorical, protective, and activist reasons. Somali American mothers in the health literacy class used the term *community sickness* to distinguish autism as a nongeneralizable experience for Somalis in diaspora, one that could not be separated out from the forced migration and ongoing structural precarity that characterized the Western diaspora. Somali American parents' "misuse" of *autism* and *community sickness* rejects the powerful discourses of medicine as capable of "explaining" their experiences and of "healing" them (Decoteau, 2021, p. 44). As agentive rhetorical refusals, Somali American students' wrong uses of *autism* and *community sickness* disrupt the top-down, abstracted model of medical disability and insist on other ways of knowing autism, disability, and sickness. Each use of *community sickness* produces meaning, disengages from medical and ableist discourses, and insists on Somali individuals' lived experiences of disability in diaspora. Referring to autism as community sickness is a rhetorical move to speak to the ways social inequality shapes the lived experience of disability, to speak to the structural, upstream causes of sickness, and to call for action that responds to these experiences, rather than for clinical tools that respond to individual bodies and their diagnoses.

Such uses of *autism* and *community sickness,* in turn, open other possibilities for action and healing. Medical diagnoses are useful to identify a condition so that clinicians can recommend a course of treatment, cure, and individual care. But this line of treatment, as becomes clear in chapter 3, was not what many participating parents were interested in when the state invited Somali parents to author their own care plans. In their definitions of autism, Somali American students spoke to the importance of supporting their children as they were. Somali American students described fears of how their Black sons would be misperceived as threats as they went about their daily lives. Students worried that a diagnosis of autism would bring surveillance and disciplinary action to their children at school. Students worried that cultural stigma surrounding disability would cut their children off from their Somali communities. Students worried about the unknown ways that forced migration was affecting the minds and bodies of their children. These were the concerns that discourses of community sickness centered. Accordingly, as chapter 3 shows in greater detail, few participating Somali American parents were interested primarily in medical forms of care—signing their children up for weekly appointments with specialists, intensive behavioral interventions, long lists of incremental goals, and new, therapeutic layers of surveillance. Rather, participants sought stable housing; educational aid for their children; reliable, affordable, and healthy food; safety; economic support as they found their footing in a new country; and connections to home and faraway kin.

Imagining what would help her, one participant, Roukia, had drawn a house with a fence on her state application for disability-related services. Like Nur, Roukia described a place where her children were not expected to exhibit a concern for property. A place that wouldn't kick her children out and fine her family each time a child expressed rage or joy too physically. Roukia did not wish to change her children, but she did want a private, comfortable refuge where they could be their own family and where they would be protected from the vectors of community sickness. By refusing a medical discourse of autism and continuing to use an erroneous, unsanctioned set of discourses, Somali American students used the levers of language to make legible a world where these supports exist. A world where sociostructural, upstream causes of health disparities are centered. A world where the stigmas and social structures that make autism disabling are targeted for change. A world where children are not surveilled and disciplined at school and in public. In short: a world where the causes of community sickness are addressed. Participating Somali American students, in using the discourses of community sickness, crafted rhetorical tools to make this world possible.

Community Sickness as Rhetorical Refusal's Fertile Ground

Somali American participants' use of the term *community sickness* surfaces the fertile ground that compelled students to reject medical models of autism as an individual, neurodevelopmental malady. Somali American parents' use of *community sickness* as rhetorical refusal demonstrates how rhetorical refusals respond to complex, structural exigences. Such exigences are often bracketed by powerful discourses in favor of technical exigences that uphold personal responsibility. When reviewing the health literacy course post-test scores and interview transcripts, the health literacy team attributed Somali students' uses of terms like *community sickness* to students' enduring low health literacy and vulnerability to disinformation. The exigence, here, is lacking health literacy, addressable through targeted health education. By contrast, Somali American participants' rhetorical refusals enacted through the discourses of *community sickness* locate exigence for dissent in a nexus of precarity—layers of stigma; pervasive ableism; the medicalization of disability; racism and racist surveillance and discipline structures in school, law enforcement, and public spaces; housing discrimination; and color-blind approaches to autism diagnosis and therapeutics.

Thus, one function of rhetorical refusal is to push against technical and individualized exigences identified as causes of noncompliance and dissent and, in turn, point to other, often obscured exigences—the more structural, embedded exigences that call for social, collective solutions. Somali American students' uses of *community sickness* show how rhetorical refusals can rewrite exigences that have been institutionally ordained and that have achieved popular consensus. One way that rhetorical refusals disrupt flows of power and discourse, then, is by responding to and making possible the recognition of obscured exigences. Rhetorical refusals insist on obscured, difficult to address, social exigences that compel dissent. For this reason, *community sickness* is an important term with which to begin this book. It gives voice to the exigences or fertile ground that sustain the rhetorical refusals described in this chapter and the following three chapters. The next chapters follow how actions—nonvaccination, not completing social service forms, and providing at-home, naturopathic care for children—both refuse medical, public health, and disability services that do not respond to community sickness and enact protection and constrained care for community sickness.

Conclusion

This chapter has engaged Somali American students' definitions of autism as community sickness. This concept—autism as community sickness—is important in two main regards. First, students' uses of *autism* as "community sickness" were rhetorical refusals, ones crafted by participants through alternative, wrong, and unsanctioned discourses. Somali American students used these discourses to describe autism on their own terms—to genealogize and personalize autism, to focus on the sociostructural causes of disability for Somali families in diaspora, and to find each other and share resources. Second, students' articulations of autism as community sickness speaks to the obscured exigences that inform these and other rhetorical refusals. Indeed, one critical function of rhetorical refusal is to insist on exigences that mainstream, dominant discourses obscure but that nonetheless shape people's health beliefs, actions, and daily lives. The next chapter considers how experiences of autism as community sickness compelled participants to use nonvaccination as a participatory mode of embodied rhetorical refusal. Somali American participants refused to prioritize vaccination as a technical solution to social problems and pushed beyond the metrics of a widely vaccinated, regularly circulating public to articulate healthy communities differently. The experience of autism as community sickness, as discussed in this chapter, informs these embodied rhetorical refusals, which arc toward different health futures.

CHAPTER 2

Outbreak

Vaccine Dissent as Embodied Rhetorical Refusal

Somali Minnesotans had been campaigning since 2006 for greater attention to what many suspected was an unexplained autism cluster among Somali American children. But it was not until mid-2017 that Somali concerns about autism gained a public, national platform—only not for reasons anyone wanted. In April 2017, Minnesotans experienced the state's largest measles outbreak since 1990. As described in this book's introduction, the outbreak primarily affected Somali Minnesotan children who had not received both doses of the MMR vaccine. As measles cases spread in the Twin Cities, as travel warnings were issued, and as daycares preventatively closed classrooms, the vaccine decisions of Somali American parents became a matter of public attention, discourse, and controversy. But Somali American parents' concerns about autism clusters extended far beyond those few, frenzied spring months in 2017. This chapter maps the public discourses documenting the 2017 measles outbreak and then turns to Somali parents' stories, which diverge from media and public health coverage and speak to the outbreak's wider contexts.

Beginning in 2006, Somali Minnesotans pressed their state to investigate why their children were overrepresented in school programs for children on the autism spectrum (MDH, 2009; Hewitt et al., 2013). It took seven years of activism, but in 2013, a research team from the University of Minnesota conducted the Minneapolis Somali Autism Spectrum Disorder Prevalence Project, which documented the racial breakdown of students enrolled in public preschool ASD (autism spectrum disorder) programs. Findings confirmed that the proportion of Somali children who participated in a preschool ASD program was higher than that of children of other racial and ethnic backgrounds. The study was not designed to investigate the reasons for these differences, but publications offered possible explanations. Perhaps, the study's community report explained, differences were a result of better outreach about preschool ASD programs to Somali families. Or maybe non-Somali children used autism services outside of the public school system more than Somali children. Or, yes, it could be that Somali children did experience higher rates of autism than other groups, for reasons unknown (Hewitt et al., 2013).

The research team also conducted a prevalence study of autism diagnosis rates among seven- to nine-year-old children living in Minneapolis. Findings showed that one in 32 Somali children were diagnosed with autism, compared to one in 36 white children in the same population segment. Statistically, there was no difference between the two rates. Also documented was a higher prevalence of autism among Somali and white children than among non-Somali African American and Hispanic children. The study also found that Somali children with autism were diagnosed with an accompanying intellectual disability at much higher rates than other children. All Somali children with autism (100%) were diagnosed with a co-occurring intellectual disability (Hewitt et al., 2013), in contrast to national rates that estimated 31% of children diagnosed with autism were also diagnosed with an intellectual disability (Maenner et al., 2021). Again, it was beyond the scope of a prevalence study to trace causation. Further, disability clusters are notoriously difficult to distinguish from chance clusters; when it comes to autism, the cause itself remains unknown, and so it is unclear what, beyond prevalence, might be worth investigating. In short, more research was needed to verify and understand the differences in prevalence of autism rates among Somali and non-Somali children.

Still, members of the research team posited interpretations in community meetings and reports. Some researchers suggested that the similar diagnosis rates between Somali and white children could be a sign of progress; because white children have historically been diagnosed with autism earlier and more accurately than their peers of color, the similar prevalence of autism diagnoses between white and Somali children could mean that Somali children were getting diagnosed earlier and with more accuracy than other children of color. Conversely, the high rates of co-occurring intellectual disability diagnoses among Somali children could be, on one hand, a fluke of a relatively small sample size or, on the other, an indication of underidentification of Somali children with autism. Perhaps practitioners were only diagnosing autism in

Somali children who were severely affected, meaning that practitioners were missing milder presentations in Somali children and that their autism rates were higher than recorded (Hewitt et al., 2016). Although there were no conclusions about how to read the results of this surveillance study, all Somali parents I spoke with identified this study as evidence that Somali children experienced inexplicably higher rates of autism and that nobody in power cared enough to investigate why. The study had done little to assuage concerns or offer answers.

Amid Somali-led calls for institutions to take their concerns seriously, leaders of antivaccination organizations visited Minneapolis and held informational meetings targeting Somali audiences (Sohn, 2017; Sun, 2017), a coordinated initiative that I discuss later in the chapter. For now, I note that the 2017 outbreak occurred when many interests and worldviews were in conflict. There were Somali American parents worried about their children's health, education, and futures. There were Somali activist groups who advocated for their concerns to be heard. There were researchers trying to make sense of autism prevalence across populations. There were antivaccination groups equipped with well-packaged answers at a time of great uncertainty. There were public health officials focused on increasing vaccination rates. And then there was an infectious disease outbreak.

This chapter maps stories of the outbreak through three different sites of outbreak discourse: news media coverage, public health accounts, and Somali Minnesotan parents' stories. This chapter begins with a historical review of US news coverage of vaccine controversy, one that charts how the wrong-belief frame came to describe all cases of vaccine hesitancy and, with it, how the white, (over)educated, privileged mother emerged as the prototypical antivaxxer (Conis, 2014; Hausman, 2019; Lawrence, 2020). In news coverage of the 2017 measles outbreak, the figure of the Somali nonvaccinator initially challenged but ultimately reaffirmed the wrong-belief frame, its stock character of the antivax mother, and its racialized and gendered assumptions about who refuses vaccines and why. Next, the chapter analyzes news and public health coverage of the outbreak. These authoritative discourses told an aligned story of two agents, public health departments and antivaccination groups, who battled over the beliefs of Somali parents. Somali parents and their decision-making were flattened into the passive grounds over which a vaccination debate was fought. This mainstream narrative differed greatly from the stories I heard in interviews with Somali parents. The second part of the chapter engages these stories. Participants' stories cohered around seven themes that point to a collective sense of exclusion from the production of medical knowledge and the benefits of medical progress. Building on the arguments parents made within these themes, I then theorize parents' vaccine dissent as rhetorical refusal, as rhetorical participation that stems from underaddressed exigences and that arcs toward different norms in clinical research and different models of community health. Parents' rhetorical refusals disrupt mainstream narratives about nonvaccination and rethink vaccine dissent, community health, and clinical research practices. Parents' rhetorical refusals work not just in a symbolic way but in an epistemic way to flag potentially real health problems and to productively contest scientific knowledge. In research on vaccine hesitancy, this epistemic function of vaccine refusal has been largely elided in a focus on either correcting vaccine refusal or reading vaccine refusal as an idiom for larger concerns. Rhetorical refusal, however, insists that audiences not only interpret the underlying contexts of vaccine refusals but listen seriously to the actual content of vaccine concerns, which can challenge science in meaningful ways.

Historical Vaccine Frames and the Rise of the Racialized Wrong-Belief Frame

Antivaccine sentiments have been around for as long as vaccines have been around (Hausman, 2019), but the journalistic frames covering vaccine dissent have been anything but stable. In this section, I summarize historical and contemporary frames used to cover vaccine controversy in news reporting. This history depicts how the wrong-belief frame and its key character, the white and privileged antivax mother, solidified as a dominant way—as well as a racialized and gendered way—of explaining vaccine dissent. This historical context shows how vaccine dissent has been rhetorically racialized and gendered in ways that both overemphasize and lambaste white mothers' concerns while silencing anyone else's vaccine concerns. The dominance of the wrong-belief frame bears specific effects for persons of color, whose vaccine dissent often stems from and surfaces racist structures in medicine (Samudzi, 2017; Goldenberg, 2021; Charles, 2022). But the wrong-belief frame focuses on the individual beliefs and, in doing so, preempts consideration of the relationship between systemic racism and vaccine dissent.

US News Media Frames for Vaccine Controversy

Historian Elena Conis's study of journalistic coverage of vaccine controversy documents how each era from the 1960s to the 2000s produced its own historically contingent interpretive frame for understanding vaccine dissent. For example, pharmaceutical marketing campaigns and popular news coverage framed the first measles vaccine as a "great equalizer," a timely sentiment that aligned with President Lyndon B. Johnson's contemporaneous war on poverty (Conis, 2014, p. 55). The mumps vaccine was positioned as a modern middle-class convenience, a technological advancement that could help mothers skip the time-consuming challenges of caring for sick children at home; this framing meshed with the era's postwar prioritization of domestic efficiency (pp. 67–70). As well, each period advanced a historically contingent explanation for vaccine dissent. In the 1960s, news accounts of outbreaks directed blame to the urban poor, a population commonly scapegoated as morally inferior vectors for disease (pp. 50–63). Blame shifted in the 1970s and 1980s to a stingy federal government that defaulted on its responsibility to make childhood vaccines accessible to everyone. Blame expanded in the 1980s and into the 2000s to include a greedy pharmaceutical industry, a broken healthcare system, and upper-class liberals (pp. 14–17). So, too, did public health invocations to parents to vaccinate their children change as different claims became persuasive at different times. Vaccine campaigns in the 1960s and 1970s broadcasted "gruesome complications" of diseases once considered mild and common, such as measles and mumps (pp. 77–85; Conis and Hoenicke, 2022). In the 2000s, as infectious diseases became much less common in the US and therefore less viscerally threatening, public health communications and outreach urged parents to uphold their social responsibility and vaccinate their children (pp. 105–111). As Conis summarizes, "the benefits of vaccination hadn't changed, but each era produced its own call to arms" (2014, p. 9).

By 2000, American news stories described vaccine dissent as sustained by maternal fears that the MMR vaccine could cause autism (Conis, 2014, pp. 203–220). This story came to dominate and homogenize news coverage of vaccine dissent. In 1998, former physician Andrew Wakefield published a fraudulent study that posited a link between the MMR vaccine and autism. The study was redacted but has continued to provoke fear and bear an outsized impact on media coverage of vaccine controversy. Conis described the pre-Wakefield turn of the century as a time when "reports about vaccine dangers became a regular feature in the news," but, notably, this coverage was evenhanded, "event-driven and diverse" (p. 204). Stories covered, for example, the briefly recalled rotavirus vaccine, parental concerns about side effects from the hepatitis B vaccine, and moderate public debate about the pros and cons of regular flu vaccination. But then, "over the course of the decade [. . .] one vaccine-safety story gradually supplemented all others: the story of the relationship between autism and vaccines" (p. 204). Conis documented that the

Wakefield controversy and MMR-autism link was mentioned in US newspapers 400 times in 2001 and more than 3,000 times in 2009 (p. 212). Had the redacted study's influence really expanded that much? Scholars have argued that the answer is no. Rather, the Wakefield study proved rhetorically useful for cementing the wrong-belief frame as the dominant frame in order to discredit all forms of vaccine doubt (Hausman, 2019, p. 32, pp. 44–48, pp. 54–59). In the wrong-belief frame, vaccine dissent is an individual problem, and it is caused by bad information. Good, scientific information elicits vaccine confidence; bad, erroneous information breeds vaccine doubts. Out was coverage that handled vaccine dissent with nuance and an attunement to local differences; in was a broad-brush approach to denigrating all vaccine doubts as wrong and an offense to science. Following Conis's historical analysis, the question remains: Why was this story a particularly kairotic one with which to explain vaccine dissent at this time? The next section takes up this question by considering the wrong-belief frame's central character, the white, affluent, panicky mother.

Race, Gender, and Motherhood in the Wrong-Belief Frame

Within the wrong-belief frame, white, privileged, Wakefield-brainwashed mothers were positioned as the prototypical antivaxxers (Conis, 2014; Hausman, 2019, pp. 36–48; Lawrence, 2020, pp. 62–73). Media coverage within the wrong-belief frame has depicted the voluntary nonvaccinator as a "misinformed, irrational, vaccine fearing parent," as "a caricature of the educated, well-off, twenty-first century parent. [. . .] She was a parent who trusted alternative medicines, organic food, and yoga" (Conis, 2014, p. 219). Antivaxxer mothers were cast as "foolish, unthinking, uncaring bimbos" (Lawrence, 2020, p. 71); they were "stupid or deluded," not only "scientifically illiterate" but "immune to convincing scientific arguments about the value of vaccination" (Hausman, 2019, p. 64; p. 33). The privileged antivax mother was dismissed as lost in an antiscience wormhole and explained away as the result of bad information. Despite the lack of evidence supporting the actual demographic prevalence of wealthy, white mothers in comparison to other vaccine dissenters (Hausman, 2019, p. 36), this character has proven rhetorically useful to discredit vaccine dissent as a hyperbolic action undertaken by unhinged mothers.

Lawrence (2020) has shown how the 2014–2015 Disneyland measles outbreak exemplifies the wrong-belief frame in action. Outbreak reporting centered blame on the choices of wealthy, white Californian mothers, known for securing vaccine exemptions that insulated their children from medical interventions while putting other children at risk of infectious disease exposure (Reich, 2014). In fall 2014 there was intensive reporting about high rates of personal belief exemptions at Los Angeles elite private schools (Lawrence, 2020, pp. 62–73; Hausman, 2019, pp. 47–50). Coverage centered on wealthy Californian antivax moms and explained that they were consumed by "a diffuse constellation of unproven anxieties, from allergies and asthma to eczema and seizure" (Khazan, 2014). *The Atlantic,* in their coverage of the outbreak, featured a stock image of a blonde woman doing yoga on a paddleboard, captioned: "If you can do yoga on a paddleboard, you can get an MMR vaccine." News coverage of the Disneyland outbreak focused blame for failures to achieve high vaccination rates, national immunity, and disease elimination on selfish mothers who secured personal belief exemptions. The proper response, then, was to tighten personal belief exemptions (Lawrence, 2020, pp. 70–73). The wrong-belief frame illustrates why, in the case of vaccination, arhetorical responses, such as mandates, are the norm (Lawrence, 2020, pp. 49–59). If nonvaccinators are entitled, rich Californians who are flat-out wrong, why spend time persuading them when you can mandate them?

Rhetorician Jordynn Jack (2014) has shown that "one way to study a rhetorical controversy is to follow the characters that appear, examining the ways they are named, invoked, and deployed by different speakers for rhetorical effect in different times and places" (p. 3). Publicly available subjectivities extend to individuals the authority to speak and be heard in the public sphere, the space of public discourse and change, and deprive others, from the start, of rhetorical ethos. The powerful subjectivity of the nutty antivax mom is particularly effective in this regard as it preemptively codes as wrong all expressions of vaccine hesitancy. The wrong-belief frame and its depiction of the antivaxxer as a spiraling white mother neutralizes a biomedical worldview and its individualistic approaches to disease management and reduces all vaccine concerns to scientific error (Leach and Fairhead, 2008). As Hausman (2019) writes of the wrong-belief frame,

> to make the argument that vaccine skepticism is a problem of belief and not, for instance, a problem of public health policy and practice, concerns about government overreach, fears about corruption in medical research and the development of pharmaceuticals, or the result of actual bad experiences with vaccination, these other possible ways of framing vaccination concerns have to be discounted or obscured. (p. 33)

The persistent framing of vaccine hesitancy as a problem of wrong parental belief shrinks the discursive tools available for making arguments about structural causes of voluntary nonvaccination, including those suggested by

Hausman above. The wrong-belief frame keeps anyone expressing any form of vaccine hesitancy rhetorically disabled from the start (Owens, 2013), as their concerns cannot be heard as anything other than error, the jabbering of a science denialist, the lost-cause wealthy mother (Hausman, 2019, pp. 87–109). The subjectivity of white, privileged mother as "premier anti-vaxxer" (Conis, 2014, p. 225) therefore keeps systems of power and expertise in place because it contains voluntary nonvaccination as an individual problem; the wrong-belief frame occludes consideration of structural causes of vaccine dissent and focuses public attention and resources on individualized approaches, such as health literacy education, mandates, and the elimination of personal exemptions (Lawrence, 2020, pp. 62–70).

But what happens when people who are not white, not privileged, or not affluent express vaccine concerns? Within the wrong-belief frame and the reign of the frenzied, antivax mother, vaccine concerns raised by people outside of this subjectivity are coded as fixable symptoms of health illiteracy and access barriers to healthcare. Their concerns are coded not as the selfish, anxious missteps of the privileged but as the uninformed or misinformed actions of the marginalized. Still, neither agency nor nuance are extended to these rhetors. Demonstrating how the wrong-belief frame also overdetermines the vaccine hesitancy of not-white, not-affluent mothers, Decoteau (2021) has explained that public health accounts of vaccine hesitancy default to two categories of dissent. First, there is the dissent of the privileged, who choose not to vaccinate. Second, there is the dissent of the marginalized, who cannot access reliable healthcare, good information, or vaccines. Perhaps they cannot regularly take their children to the pediatrician, or perhaps they do not have enough understanding of basic healthcare to stay on top of vaccine schedules. No matter, their patchy vaccine records are not their own fault but reflect the barriers that poor and under-resourced people encounter. As Decoteau writes,

> Whereas whites are blamed for their vaccine decisions, marginalized populations are represented as incapable of vaccine decision-making. Public health experts draw a stark line between those who are *un*vaccinated and who consciously choose to be exempt from vaccination (generally from wealthy white neighborhoods) and those who are simply *under* vaccinated (generally poor, marginalized communities who face access and knowledge barriers). (p. 157)

As this unvaccinated and undervaccinated binary makes clear, the wrong-belief frame restricts agentive vaccine refusal to white, wealthy mothers, even as it makes fun of their deluded decision-making. In doing so, this popular frame relegates nonvaccination by other mothers as a reaction to circumstance.

Much of the qualitative research on vaccine hesitancy has focused on the views of white, affluent mothers (Lawrence, Hausman, and Dannenberg, 2014; Reich, 2014; Reich, 2016; Kolodziejski, 2020, Voyles, 2020), meaning there is little research that addresses vaccine hesitancy outside of privileged stances (with key exceptions: Charles, 2018; Charles, 2022; Thornton and Reich, 2022). Stories of bad information, predatory antivax groups, and access barriers fill in for first-person accounts of vaccine decision-making.[1] However, there is a deeply researched record of medical racism in the US and its endemic neglect of the health of Black Americans alongside the biomedical oversurveillance and abuse of Black people, a long-standing reality that Alondra Nelson (2011) has termed a "dialectic of neglect and surveillance" (p. 164), and Benjamin (2016) has theorized as "the deadly intersection of medical abandonment and overexposure" (p. 971). And yet, rarely is medical racism considered as an exigence of vaccine hesitancy. Sociologist Zoe Samudzi (2017) has written that the equating of "vaccine skeptic" with "white anti-vaxxers" who "cite scientific empirics claiming causal relationships between measles, mumps, and rubella vaccine sequences and autism diagnosis" obscures the "more complicated" and "deep-rooted" vaccine skepticism "that exists within Black communities [. . . which] stems partially from a fear of historical trauma and scientific racism that is tragically verifiable" (para. 2). Too, the wrong-belief frame and its subjectivity of the white antivax mother does not contend with the argument that just because white, affluent, and educated parents might be the most vocal about their vaccine reservations does not mean that they are the most vaccine-hesitant. It means they have the least to lose in voicing their concerns. People in more precarious positions might hold back because they have less resources to maneuver through bureaucratic processes like claiming a vaccine exemption (Hausman 2019, p. 34) or because they fear that parental behavior against public health recommendations might activate child protective services (Thornton and Reich, 2022). However, the wrong-belief frame silences the vaccine hesitancy of persons of color and persons of lower socioeconomic statuses by preemptively coding their nonvaccination as an unintentional, circumstantial response to access barriers and to bad information.

Although beyond the scope of this study's US context, the wrong-belief frame and its racialized subjectivities extend to how vaccine hesitancy in the global South has been explained. Western approaches to vaccine resistance in the global South attribute vaccine dissent to poverty, lack of access to medicine, and medical illiteracy, as well as to traditional cultural and religious

---

1. Refer to Hausman, 2019, pp. 74–86, for an analysis of Eula Biss's book *On Immunity* (2014) as an example of the presentation of Black mothers as the subjects of others' vaccine decisions and never as the agents of their own decisions.

beliefs and the pervasiveness of rumor (Leach and Fairhead, 2007)—and rarely to people's own agentive decision-making. To this point, few Western accounts of vaccine hesitancy in Africa begin with the rich history of African variolation practices; most Western accounts identify vaccination as a new technology brought by European and American colonizers. But successful variolation infrastructures were in place across Africa before colonial powers dismissed these practices and instituted their own vaccination regimes (Waite, 1987; White, 2000). Colonial medical documentarians ignored African variolation practices, but, tellingly, colonial public health officials' ledgers noted that the East African communities known for being the most resistant to smallpox vaccination were also those with the most widespread variolation practices, always "without drawing any inference as to why" (White, 2000, p. 289). There was no consideration that Africans might resist a colonizer's vaccine because they were already vaccinated; rather, resistance was attributed to poor understandings of science and susceptibility to superstition. An entire continent's science and practices of immunization were recorded as a lack.

Somali Minnesotans, as refugees from East Africa who, in the US, are marginalized by race, ethnicity, gender, religion, and class, speak from positions of multiple marginalities. Medical, public health, and mainstream audiences often hear Somalis' vaccine hesitancies as unfortunate effects of scientific illiteracy, poverty, the experience of living in nations with poor healthcare infrastructure, and premodern cultural and religious beliefs. However, when Somali American parents' nonvaccination practices became matters of public concern during the 2017 measles outbreak, Somali Americans' nonvaccination practices found brief traction to disrupt these power-produced and -producing narratives about agency, science, history, and race. Because the wrong-belief frame relied on the figure of the worried-well mother sending herself down antivax wormholes, this frame could not be seamlessly ported over to cover the 2017 measles outbreak, where Somali parents were the ones declining vaccines. New stories were necessary. But, as the remainder of this chapter shows, there was only a brief window wherein Somali Americans' embodied vaccine refusals were legible to broader publics before the wrong-belief frame closed back in.

The wrong-belief frame and its attendant subjectivity of the privileged, white antivax mother, useful to explain (away) vaccine dissent, continued to shape news coverage of and public health responses to the 2017 Minnesota outbreak. Coverage of the 2017 outbreak briefly fractured but ultimately cohered within the comprehensive wrong-belief frame. The outbreak, then, is both an example of the durability of the wrong-belief frame and a depiction of the uneven, power-consolidated rhetorical terrain in which Somali American mothers, as marginalized rhetors, vie to speak and often get ignored, misunderstood, and explained away. For these reasons, Somali American rhetorical vaccine refusals, addressed in the second half of this chapter, are urgent and power-disrupting.

"When Anti-Vaxxers Target Immigrants": News Narratives of the Minnesota Measles Outbreak

Local and national reporting of the Minnesota measles outbreak circulated a common story: antivaccination groups identified Somali Minnesotans as a vulnerable population whose autism concerns made them amenable to antivaccination arguments and then targeted them with disinformation campaigns that lowered Somali vaccination rates and left everyone, and Somali American children especially, vulnerable to infectious disease. The *Washington Post* attributed agency to antivaccination groups in the headline, "Antivaccine Activists Spark a State's Worst Measles Outbreak in Decades" (Sun, 2017). CBS Minnesota advanced a similar narrative: "State health officials said the Somali community has been targeted with misinformation about the dangers of vaccines" (Wagner, 2017). Fox News echoed: "Minnesota Measles Outbreak: Officials Say Somali Families 'Targeted with Misinformation'" (Chamberlain, 2017). Minnesota's *Star Tribune* ran the headline "Antivaccine Groups Step Up Outreach to Minnesota Somali Families over Measles Outbreak" (Howatt and Mahamud, 2017). Science news publication *Stat News* reported in kind: "Measles Sweeps an Immigrant Community Targeted by Antivaccine Activists" (Branswell, 2017).

Opinion pieces published in the wake of the outbreak kept this narrative alive. *Mic*'s post-outbreak assessment was delivered under the headline "Anti-Vaxxers 'Targeted' Minnesota's Somali Community: Now They Have a Measles Outbreak" (Swartz, 2017). *Wired* condensed the outbreak story for its readers: "Anti-Vaxxers Brought Their War to Minnesota—Then Came Measles" (Molteni, 2017). *Vox*'s longform coverage was titled "Minnesota's Measles Outbreak Is What Happens When Anti-Vaxxers Target Immigrants" (Belluz, 2017); the article summarized the outbreak's catalyst:

> In 2008, antivaccine advocates—including the Organic Consumers Association and Andrew Wakefield, a British doctor who falsified data suggesting vaccines are linked to autism—began targeting local Somali Americans who had concerns about autism among their children. The activists saw an opening, offering an explanation when the health department couldn't provide

one. Vaccination rates plummeted in the community over the next several years, making its members more susceptible to preventable diseases such as measles and mumps.

Such narratives characterized Somali Minnesotan parents as afraid, "marginalized," and "vulnerable," emphasized their lack of English language proficiency and scientific literacy, and described how antivaccine groups "targeted" Somalis' fear and lack of medical knowledge. Molteni's narrative summary is representative: "Over the last decade, anti-vaxxers have fortified this corner of Minneapolis into a bastion for pseudo-science. It all began with higher-than-normal rates of severe autism in the Somali community. [. . .] In came the anti-vax partisans, whose success with these frightened parents has turned the neighborhood into a beachhead for what should be a preventable disease." These news and opinion stories are, on one hand, accurate and important. Many Somali Minnesotan parents did have concerns about their children's vulnerability to autism. National antivaccination organizations did descend on Minneapolis, did set up shop in Somali community spaces, and did deliver disinformation about unsubstantiated links between the MMR vaccine and autism. But these narratives also automatically position Somali American parents as the passive recipients of antivaccine information and never as the active decoders, assemblers, and localizers of different types of information to meet their needs. These narratives locate the seed of vaccine hesitancy in disinformation and never in broader contexts that might compel distrust in medicine, public health, and institutional expertise, never in the fertile ground that might make antivaccination logical or protective.

Some uncommon narratives told in news coverage of the measles outbreak offer glimpses of the stories left out of this dominant narrative. Sun (2017) reported on Somali-led pro-vaccine activism and described collaborations with imams and public health officials to provide families with resources, like transportation, to get their children vaccines. This reporting fragmented the singular narrative that Somali Americans were victims of disinformation campaigns. Other journalists reported on Somali leaders' comments that there was more to the measles outbreak than the targeted deliverance of disinformation to an ill-informed, insular public. Arthur Nazaryan, reporting on Public Radio Exchange, centered the voices of Somali Minnesotans who explained that persisting health disparities and a long-standing lack of relationship with public health helped fuel the outbreak. Activist Abdirizak Bihi explained that the most pressing problem was a "lack of education about how to engage the health care system on the patient side, and a lack of cultural awareness on the provider side. It's a gap in understanding [. . .] that public health officials used to fill fairly well on a local level—but no longer do" (as qtd. in Nazaryan, 2017). Bihi's explanation described interlocking causes of the outbreak and pointed to a series of relational breakdowns between Somalis and public health workers, all happening within an underfunded public health system. This explanation directs attention to the ways that interpersonal trust is built and eroded through relationships and away from questions of scientific literacy and information transmission. While these alternative stories did not deny the influence of antivaccination disinformation campaigns, they did allow for more complex causal narratives. In these stories, there appeared pro-vaccine Somali groups collaborating with public health workers to inculcate vaccine trust, and there emerged disillusioned Somali Minnesotans using their own experiences, not just disinformation funneled to them, to decide whether to trust public health recommendations. Still, it was the story of powerful antivaccination groups preying on vulnerable Somalis that took hold as the explanatory narrative of the outbreak, not only in news coverage but also in public health explanations of the outbreak, as the next section describes.

"There's Nothing Wrong with Them": Public Health Narratives of the Minnesota Measles Outbreak

Public health reports also depicted Somali American parents as a vulnerable public taken advantage of by antivaccination groups. Public health statements condemned the influence of antivaccine arguments and claimed that public health as an institution should have executed more culturally sensitive vaccination campaigns. A paper by Minnesota Department of Health (MDH) epidemiologists and public health experts concluded that an enduring challenge for Minnesota's public health workers was outreach to their Somali community members; the authors wrote, "Although MDH, LPH, and community partners have done outreach work with the Somali Minnesotan community since 2008, the fear of autism and the active involvement of antivaccination groups to spread misinformation about MMR vaccines continue to undermine public health efforts" (Banerjee et al., 2020, p. 163). The authors concluded that "partnerships between public health, health care providers and influential community and religious leaders are critical in addressing vaccine misinformation, resulting in increased trust, which can lead to higher immunization rates and compliance with public health interventions" (p. 170). Other public health reports recommended similar culturally specific outreach, including "outreach to community leaders, parents, interpreters, and spiritual leaders to provide information on vaccines and vaccine preventable diseases" because "encouraging medical providers to use interpreters, take time to build trust, and assess vaccination status at every visit might improve vaccination coverage in these populations" (Leeds and Muscoplat, 2017). These takeaways square with a culture-based approach to noncompliance; these remarks delineate that disinformation stokes vaccine hesitancy and that culturally specific outreach and the dissemination of scientifically sound information can combat hesitancy and increase compliance.

Accordingly, state public health responses to the outbreak focused on efforts to get, first, vaccines and, later, information to Somali Minnesotans. Upon the identification of the first two measles cases, public health interventions began immediately and continued around the clock. MDH sought to quickly reach Somali populations and rapidly administer post-exposure prophylactic vaccinations (Hall et al., 2017). MDH worked with local partners, including local public health agencies, healthcare facilities, childcare centers, schools, and Somali community partners, to investigate cases, confirm cases with laboratory testing, conduct contact tracing, administer prophylactic treatments to those without immunity, and implement quarantines (Banerjee et al., 2020). By May 31, 2017, at least 154 persons had taken a post-exposure prophylactic vaccination. The average number of MMR vaccine doses administered per week in Minnesota increased from 2,700 doses before the outbreak to 9,964 by mid-May (Hall et al., 2017). The 586 exposed persons who did not receive a post-exposure vaccination quarantined (Hall et al., 2017). A year after the measles outbreak, vaccination rates in Minnesota increased 16 percentage points among children of Somali descent (Richert, 2018).

MDH also hosted community educational events, shared information with Somali community and faith leaders, and disseminated educational information via Somali media outlets. MDH established an information hotline where 200 callers could simultaneously listen to a physician report on the dangers of measles and the importance of vaccination (Richert, 2018). The hotline not only provided an efficient means of distributing information but was also attuned to Somali preferences for oral communication (Banerjee et al., 2020). Public health authorities coordinated outreach efforts that translated their materials into Somali and Oromo languages, incorporated stories to illustrate otherwise decontextualized facts, and tapped into oral channels of communication through radio, video streaming, and on-site engagement. Inclusion efforts involved hiring Somali staff to serve as outreach coordinators and interpreters and ensuring that Somali interpreters were available at all county clinics (Hall et al., 2017; Richert, 2018). Director of Infectious Disease Epidemiology, Prevention and Control Division at MDH Kristin Ehresmann explained that after the outbreak, MDH prioritized hiring Somali staff for community engagement positions: "We have one Somali outreach worker whose job it is to make sure parents are aware of resources they can have for their children if they do have [autism] concerns. Then we have an outreach worker who is focused on providing information on immunizations" (as qtd. in Belluz, 2017). During the outbreak, Hennepin County Health Department and the health insurance company Allina deployed Allina's Somali-speaking staff to disseminate the county's pro-vaccination message. MDH assembled a team of Somali medical professionals, faith leaders, elected officials, and community leaders to distribute MDH-authored educational materials at community events, childcare centers, schools, and mosques (Banerjee et al., 2020). These efforts prioritized developing culturally attuned methods of health education for Somali people in Minnesota.

Public health responses to the Minnesota measles outbreak were effective in that public health quickly identified and responded to the outbreak, identified cases, tracked cases, delivered treatments, and contained the outbreak with no fatalities. This is a huge feat. At the same time, post-outbreak public health responses focused on getting information to Somali Minnesotans in culturally appropriate and persuasive ways. This response adhered to the assumption that Somali parents were "under vaccinated" and not "unvaccinated" (Decoteau, 2021, p. 157). As medical sociologist Donna McAlpine described, "There's nothing wrong with them. There's something wrong with us [public health]" (as qtd. in Bellware, 2017). Public health responses laudably contained outbreak and increased vaccination rates, but they did not, as I show in the rest of the chapter, necessarily respond to Somali American parents' concerns. Thus, Somali trust in vaccination remained tenuous.

The Wrong-Belief Frame in the Minnesota Measles Outbreak

News and public health accounts of the 2017 outbreak could not rely on the wrong-belief frame and its subjectivity of the privileged white mother because in this outbreak, it was the Somali mother who was opting out of childhood vaccines. In response, news and public health accounts described the Somali nonvaccinating parent as a victim of scientific illiteracy and targeted disinformation campaigns. Across published accounts of the 2017 measles outbreak, the vulnerable, ill-informed, and duped Somali parent arose as a secondary kind of antivaxxer: the blameless, reformable antivaxxer. This character was distinct from the privileged white mother, but both subjectivities were harnessed to advance the individualistic wrong-belief frame of nonvaccination. Demonstrating the power of the wrong-belief frame as well as the enduring culpability of the white, privileged mother and the emergent passivity of the nonwhite mother, health reporter Beth Mole's account of the Minnesota measles outbreak is illustrative:

> In the past, the Somali community had some of the highest vaccination rates in the state. But with deep-seated fears of autism and a—now debunked—rumor that autism rates were rising in their community, many fell victim to the misinformation spread by local and national antivaccination advocates. Those include notorious antivaccine advocate Andrew Wakefield, a fraudulent former physician stripped of his medical credentials for falsifying data, abusing children, and other professional misconduct. Health experts did not shy away from pinpointing the local problem: "It's white, middle-class parents who have made a decision not to vaccinate and feel very strongly about that choice," Kris Ehresmann, director of infectious disease epidemiology at the Minnesota Department of Health, told the *Post*. (Mole, 2017)

In this summary, the selfish white mother remained the prototypical vaccine refuser. Somali parents remained blameless but also voiceless. Relieved of responsibility, the Somali mother was also relieved of agency. Her own decision-making processes, prior knowledge, experiential expertise, concerns, and expectations were overwritten with forgivable ignorance. She was not senselessly "unvaccinated"; she was reversibly "under vaccinated" (Decoteau, 2021, p. 157). When the Somali parent entered the wrong-belief framework, the wrong beliefs were not the Somali parent's fault, but they were still wrong beliefs. Wrong beliefs could be corrected by better, more culturally appropriate information. This narrative kept the focus on personal belief, bracketed discussion of nonvaccination as structural, and redirected attention from upstream causes of medical dissent.

But other stories pushed against this comprehensive stock story (Martinez, 2020). Somali American mothers' nonvaccination was a rhetorical response—an embodied rhetorical refusal—articulated within this deterministic, silencing narrative. Somali American mothers, as marginalized rhetors whose vaccine doubts, in spaces of public and expert discourse, were adroitly explained away as symptoms of illiteracy, used other rhetorical modes to participate in public discourse about vaccination. Parents crafted constrained, embodied rhetorical refusals to disrupt the wrong-belief frame and its atomizing focus on personal beliefs. These rhetorical refusals responded to embodied, social, and historical exigences and arc toward different relationships between public health and the publics of public health. The chapter next turns to Somali American parents' stories of the 2017 outbreak.

Somali Stories of the Minnesota Measles Outbreak

Somali American parents' stories of the 2017 outbreak defy the wrong-belief frame. This section centers stories shared in 24 interviews I conducted with Somali parents who experienced the 2017 measles outbreak. It is structured by seven themes that emerged across interviews; these themes trace Somali parents' vaccine decisions back to lived experiences of migration, resettlement, racism, and uncertain health futures and forward toward protected children and healthy communities. Somali American parents' acts of nonvaccination, contextualized in their stories, take shape as rhetorical refusal. These rhetorical refusals are embodied and constrained; they occur in spaces where parents' voices are edged out by mainstream stories about vaccine controversies and by overdetermined rhetorical subjectivities. But, as rhetorical refusals, they interrupt, they make meaning, they protect, and they participate. Embodied rhetorical refusals enact resistance, proffer in-group somatic protection, and envision futures for community health and clinical research.

Theme 1: Experiential Endorsements of Vaccination

Although most Somali American interview participants (17 out of 24) had declined or delayed a vaccine for at least one of their children, all 24 Somali American mothers interviewed identified vaccines as lifesaving medical tools. Sixteen participants grounded their faith in vaccines in direct or secondhand experience with infectious disease outbreaks. Participants distinguished themselves from US-born Americans because their vaccine decisions were guided by their firsthand knowledge of both infectious disease and the benefits of vaccination, while their born-and-raised US counterparts were more likely to unscrupulously accept a medical provider's instruction to get whatever vaccine at whatever time. In this equation, it was the trusting American patient who was less informed, albeit docile, about disease and vaccines. Dehka, a mother of three who came to the US from Somalia in 2005, explained, "In the US, people don't get measles. But I've seen it, everyone has seen it. In rural parts of Somalia, vaccines aren't [administered . . .] and children and adults can get very sick" (3/1/2018). Sahra also expressed frustration at the perception that Somali parents were ill-informed, specifically because Somalis likely had more experience with vaccine-preventable diseases than their critics:

> I'm angry. I've seen what measles can do to children. The people saying these things, white people who have no clue, they don't know what measles is, they

don't understand vaccines. They just do what their doctor says. I know vaccines can save people. I also know that some babies shouldn't get vaccines when they're so young, some have allergies. (4/30/2018)

Kowsar, after also relating that she knew children who had been sickened by measles, advanced a similar argument: "Here, people just do what they are told, they don't know much, they don't ask questions, they take antibiotics, vaccines, Tylenol, ADHD [pharmaceuticals], whatever they're told. I think there are better ways to go through a sickness. Sometimes a vaccine is the way to go, but not always. In Africa, we were vaccinated" (4/30/2018). Kowsar's statement implies that real health literacy comes from lived experiences with disease and illness caretaking. Dehka, Sahra, and Kowsar did not come to trust vaccines because of abstract evidence or a doctor's recommendation but because of their own experiences. They knew, firsthand, the alternative to a widely vaccinated population.

Dehka's, Sahra's, and Kowsar's claims show how all three mothers drew on their experiential knowledge of infectious disease to make pro-vaccine decisions and drew on their experiential knowledge of how American healthcare affected their children's bodies to make noncompliant vaccination decisions, including decisions not to vaccinate or to spread out vaccinations. All three mothers determined that getting a child vaccinated was the right decision sometimes, but not all the time. Sahra explained that she vaccinated her children because she had experienced the dangers of infectious disease and the protective qualities of vaccination; she also vaccinated her children on a spread-out schedule because she trusted her perceptions that vaccines could have adverse effects if given to children too early in life. As Sahra's words demonstrate, many participants endorsed vaccines in general but viewed each vaccination decision as child- and situation-specific. When it came to their children's situations, Somali American parents had little faith that public health and medicine had the appropriate evidence or the appropriate level of concern for Somali American children's well-being. As a result, parents like Sahra and Kowsar turned to their own experiential knowledge and sometimes considered nonvaccination or selective or spread-out vaccination as the best strategy to protect their children's underprioritized health.

Theme 2: Situational Vaccine Decision-Making

As theme 1 demonstrated, Somali American participants rarely related to vaccination as a singular decision, to vaccines as good or bad, safe or unsafe, scientifically vetted or corrupt. Rather, participants made each vaccine decision independently. Participants' accounts of how their vaccination decisions changed in response to the measles outbreak illustrate this kind of situational vaccine decision-making in action and demonstrate how a health crisis can alter specific practices without destabilizing larger health beliefs. Eight participants reported that they vaccinated their children during the 2017 measles outbreak but that they would hesitate before continuing to vaccinate their children or vaccinating a younger child.[2] While public health accounts documented an influx in Somali vaccination rates during the measles outbreak and a steady increase in the two years following (Hall et al., 2017; Richert, 2018), interviews from my study suggest that quantitative evidence of increased vaccination rates cannot necessarily be read as evidence of changed vaccination beliefs or increased vaccine confidence. To this point, Amina, a parent who vaccinated her young child during the measles outbreak, described feeling as if she were "jumping from one fire to another" (3/2/2018). Fatouma recalled anxiously watching her newly vaccinated son for any sign of change (3/23/2018). Amina and Fatouma chose to vaccinate their children to protect them from measles during an outbreak, but their experiences with vaccination did not leave them feeling confident about their decisions. Kowsar reflected on her decision to vaccinate her three-year-old son by concluding, "My son was ok. He didn't change, so we were lucky" (3/2/2018). Even positive experiences with vaccination like Kowsar's did not undermine a larger belief system that American vaccinations were risky for Somali American children.

Amina's, Fatouma's, and Kowsar's postvaccination uneasiness reflects a pattern across interviews: Even as all 24 interviewed parents endorsed vaccines as good, every parent also discussed childhood vaccination as a weighty choice between disease risk and vaccine injury risk. No participant waived vaccination off as a standard practice, as an obvious and low- or no-risk medical event their children would undergo. Of the 24 participants who averred vaccines worked, eight also said that they believed the medical evidence supporting the safety of vaccines may not apply to Somali American individuals. Twelve participants thought it likely that certain children could be allergic to vaccines. Fourteen participants thought it likely that the MMR vaccine could cause autism in certain situations. These seemingly divergent claims suggest that Somali American parents valued vaccines in general as safe and necessary but still considered vaccination a personal decision and one for which Somali American children faced greater risks.

As a result, some Somali American parents crafted their own vaccination schedules and made vaccine decisions child by child, situation by situation.

---

2. For a closer discussion of this data, refer to Campeau (2019).

Anab described bringing together her experiences of vaccination in Africa and the US to devise her own vaccine schedule: "Lots of people think that immunizations cause this [autism], so, I said, we are going to do this differently. Less immunizations, and more spread out. [...] In Africa, they don't get so many immunizations. Here, there's hepatitis before they've left the hospital" (4/8/2018). Anab's account depicts a decision-maker who has consulted her own sources, including CDC vaccine schedules, African vaccination norms, local advice, and her own feelings. Anab's decision-making demonstrates a trust in her intuition and an adaptive response to making consequential decisions with limited information. Such ambivalence and resourcefulness suggest that participants were not against vaccination. Nor were participants uninformed about vaccination, as the news and public health accounts often assumed. Participants made involved, situation-specific vaccination choices. As anthropologists Emily Wentzell and Ana Racila have argued, "vaccine hesitancy is not a fixed trait but a calculation someone makes about the perceived risks of vaccination versus disease in a specific social and structural context" (2021, p. 245). In this study, some Somali American parents avoided the MMR vaccine when risk was low, but when measles contraction became imminent, many recalculated. Participants' practices defied categorization as either antivaccination or pro-vaccination but demonstrated ongoing and heterodox negotiations of personalized risk calculations made within unequitable healthcare systems. Parents described feeling like they could not trust population-level medical evidence or public health guidance to understand, prioritize, and therefore be relevant to their children's specific health needs. Nonvaccination emerged as a makeshift protection, necessary in a world where trust in expertise is potentially dangerous. But if Somali American parents generally trusted vaccines and the science behind vaccines, what specific risks concerned parents? What were the harms from which parents were protecting their children? The following themes address these questions.

Theme 3: Distrust of Racially Exclusive Evidence

One reason that participants wondered if vaccines might be safe for children in general but not Somali American children was what participants saw as the racially exclusive nature of evidence supporting vaccine safety. Participants doubted that clinical evidence corresponded to their embodied experiences as refugees. Twelve participants grounded their decisions to forego or delay the MMR vaccine in concerns that clinical evidence did not derive from embodied experiences of war, displacement, and resettlement. Kadra expressed her struggle to accept scientific evidence as relevant to her experience:

> I know there are studies that say vaccines do not cause autism, but they haven't done studies on us. Our children have been immunized more than American children. With my son, he had three rounds of measles immunizations. So, I want a study. Take a group of Somali children who have been vaccinated and a group that are not, and study the autism rates. I think that would tell us a lot. (4/7/2018)

Kadra was not persuaded by existing scientific evidence because such evidence did not come from research undertaken on the health of Somali refugees. Kadra also pointed to one concrete reason that Somali individuals may experience different reactions to standard vaccination: without vaccine records on hand, refugees might receive duplicate or triplicate vaccinations at refugee camps and upon resettlement. Kowsar echoed this concern and, like Kadra, envisioned research that responded to the somatic experiences of forced migration:

> We are very in support of vaccinations. Did you know that Somali children were the most vaccinated here? But we're also the most autism cases. Here's something that people don't talk about: In Africa, we were vaccinated, and we have to get vaccines in refugee camps, too. Then, we come here, we don't have vaccination records, we get vaccinated again. (3/23/2018)

Studies of refugee health align with Kadra's and Kowsar's accounts of how displaced persons are sometimes revaccinated at refugee camps and upon resettlement (Mipatrini et al., 2017). The CDC has stated that there is little risk, beyond momentary discomfort, in receiving multiple rounds of a vaccine (Moro et al., 2019). Still, Kowsar's and Kadra's experiences left both women feeling that their lived experiences did not inform the CDC's vaccination schedules.[3] Neither mother was willing to trust such generalized knowledge. In this context, nonvaccination was a form of protection that parents offered their children, one that responded to the experience of having distinct health histories not represented in clinical evidence or public health policy.

---

3. Somali mothers' insistence that their children had already been vaccinated, coupled with public health assurances that additional vaccinations would not cause harm, harken back to colonial vaccination campaigns across Africa in the early twentieth century. As discussed in the introduction, White's (2000) historical research has shown that the strongest resistance to smallpox vaccination campaigns occurred in East African communities that had their own variolation practices. But in the colonizing state's records, African variolation didn't count. Across White's historical accounts and Kowsar's and Kadra's concerns, there is a consistent dismissal of African healthcare and African people's own knowledge of their bodies and health histories. There remains resistance to regard any other pathway to immunity except for the CDC vaccination schedule and documentation of its completion.

Theme 4: Flexible Immunity

A second reason that some participants distrusted CDC vaccination schedules was that vaccination did not mesh with participants' belief systems about immunity; participants often described healthy immunity as achieved through encounters with illness followed by restorative care. This view of immunity is not unique to Somali participants. Anthropologist Emily Martin (1994) developed the concept of flexible immunity to describe a mid-twentieth-century shift in popular metaphors about immunity; popular understandings shifted from immunity as the body's defense system to immunity as a flexible system, responsive and iteratively cultivated by encounters with its environment, including with diseases (p. 37). This metaphor affects how people care for their bodies and what they expect of medicine. Personalized medicine gels with flexible immunity, but one-size-fits-all vaccines and vaccination schedules do not (Hausman, 2017). Indeed, research on vaccine hesitancy has shown that the idea of flexible immunity supports vaccine doubts. Lawrence, Hausman, and Dannenberg (2014) have identified belief in flexible immunity as informing mid-Atlantic parents' decision to forego school-sponsored flu shots. The authors described their participants' nonvaccination practices as grounded in a belief that responsible care of the immune system entailed exposure to antigens like germs and dirt. Hausman (2017), reporting on findings from an interview study of vaccine-hesitant parents living in a rural Appalachian town, also found that parents' antivaccination beliefs were influenced by flexible immunity; parents described ensuring that their children played in mud and rain and performed farm chores, tasks they saw as enriching their children's immunity and overall health (p. 295). Somali participants expressed a similar understanding of the immune system as contextual and nimble.

Distinctly, though, participating Somali parents coarticulated notions of flexible immunity with accounts of their experiences of warfare, famine, and forced migration, with recollections of healthcare procedures in Somalia, and with ambivalence about American health mandates. Anab described the differences she had experienced between the administration of vaccines in Somalia and the United States: "In Africa, there are lots of sicknesses, but not so many vaccines. Cholera, malaria. We get them, and our bodies respond. Here, we need to know whose bodies can respond and whose cannot. This affects everyone because we can't give all babies the same immunizations at the same time" (4/8/2018). In line with the theory of flexible immunity, Anab described disease not as an external threat to be controlled and eliminated but as a fortifying part of life. Also in Anab's statement, Somali people's immune systems had generationally adapted to disease rather than inoculation, and so Somali children living in Western countries might not benefit from all vaccines. Seen as flexible, personal, and shaped through lived experience, the immune system of a Somali child uprooted from home and relocated to Minneapolis would be quite different from that of a child born in the Twin Cities.

On one hand, these descriptions of the immune system depict the prevalence of flexible immunity as a health belief system; Baltimore residents (Martin, 1994), rural homesteader parents (Hausman, 2017), mid-Atlantic public-school parents (Lawrence, Hausman, and Dannenberg, 2014), and Somali parents resettled in Minnesota all articulated a similar belief in flexible immunity. On the other hand, Somali participants' uses of flexible immunity showed that their experiences as refugees and as racialized people in the US shaped their uptake of flexible immunity in nongeneralizable ways. Anab adapted a general theory of flexible immunity to argue that the lived experiences of displacement, resettlement, and structural precarity had marked her immune system in important and yet-to-be-understood ways. Positioning themselves first and foremost as Somali refugees, participants like Anab described their children's immune systems as derived from different environments and accustomed to different types of illnesses and caregiving than those of American-born children. Participants' use of flexible immunity therefore reflects the growing prevalence of the idea of flexible immunity *and* calls attention to the ways that experiences of migration, racialization, and precarity shape how many people understand the makeup of their bodies and the role medicine can play in their lives. The next three themes further engage how Somali American parents centered their positions as refugees and as marginalized people in their vaccine decision-making processes.

Theme 5: Slow Care for Illness

Some participating parents drew on the theme of flexible immunity to advocate for the healthfulness of letting children get sick and caring for sickness at home. These parents described vaccination as an unhealthful shortcut that served not public and personal health but a Western, capitalist drive to keep bodies healthy enough to go to work and school, to keep bodies circulating and producing. Some participants used nonvaccination as an embodied critique of and protection against American valuations of control and productivity. Somali American parents' nonvaccination, described thusly, can be read less as a rejection of vaccines themselves and more as a disengagement that acts in service of a world that supports rest and care.

Illustrative of this mode of vaccine dissent, Fatima echoed Anab's appreciation of sickness as a condition that strengthened immunity. Fatima then explained that she was concerned about the number of vaccines required for children in the US: "In Africa, vaccination was your choice. That's a big difference. There were less vaccines, too, and kids would get sick, they would rest, and then they would get stronger. There wasn't so much control" (3/23/2018). Fatima balked at the Western medical orientation to control and eliminate disease. Sickness was an experience that, if supported with rest, could strengthen the body. Hodan, too, critiqued vaccines as part of a medico-industrial society aimed at keeping people working rather than supporting people's long-term health. Hodan explained that she had never been against vaccines but that she had nonetheless adopted a delayed and selective vaccination schedule for her children:

> Mothers will give their children antibiotics just so the fever goes away, then send them back to daycare. There's no time to recover at home. Have a fever? Tylenol so they can go back to school. Have a virus? Antibiotics so they'll be better in two days. And they use vaccines as much as they can, even for the flu, so they don't get sick. But a few kids will have side effects from those vaccines. Just like they'll have side effects to antibiotics, Ritalin, the list goes on. (2/14/2018)

Neither Fatima nor Hodan equated a widely vaccinated and disease-free population with a healthy population. Rather, Fatima and Hodan described healthy people as those whose immune systems had grown stronger through interactions with naturally occurring disease. Both mothers saw value in illness (Hausman, 2019, p. 197; pp. 201–212); illness could make a body stronger, and illness called for care and for a family to turn inward and nurse those in need. Fatima and Hodan accordingly wondered to what extent vaccines supplanted the slow and inefficient but life-giving work of care and rest. Anab, Fatima, and Hodan were not rejecting vaccines so much as an American drive to restore health just enough so that people could reenter public, productive spaces (work, school, daycare).[4] Their selective nonvaccination opted out of American work systems that demanded disease-free, healthy-enough, circulating, and maximally productive bodies.

Indeed, children are vaccinated not only to protect them individually from disease but also to "protect their communities from disease, and the state and nation from the medical and economic burdens of disease" (Conis, 2014, p. 11). For these reasons, vaccination is a rare but "key health citizenship

---

4. Refer also to Hausman (2019, pp. 208–212) for interpretation of vaccine resistance as a resistance to "modernity and its reliance on the circulation of people, goods, and money in modern economies" (p. 209).

responsibility of children" (Conis, 2014, p. 11). Anab's, Fatima's, and Hodan's expressions of vaccine dissent were expressions of skepticism regarding the potential prioritization of protection of the state and its economic productivity over the protection of children, especially racialized children, whose health, Somali American mothers knew firsthand, was not the state's top priority. These mothers did not buy into this expected form of health citizenship. They were questioning the operationalization of vaccines to serve Western goals of productivity, control over disease, and economic circulation. They were wondering if their children might bear disproportionate burdens in this civic responsibility. Few participants in this study felt they could trust state-sanctioned views of bodies, health, and risk. Informed by lived experiences of racism and being rendered expendable, Fatima's, Hodan's, and Anab's rejections of the community protection offered by vaccines were enactments of a differently bounded kind of protection for their children. They delineated Somali children as the biosocial public they sought to protect. To do so, they made health decisions that were not in the best interest of the public. Vaccine refusals were efforts to protect their children in state systems that demanded equal participation but that did not provide equal protection. Vaccine refusals were efforts to protect their children's abilities to rest and recover, their family's ability to give and receive care, to respond to the body's needs and unpredictable timelines. Their generative refusals acted in the service of a world where there was time for care, rest, and slow healing.

Theme 6: Protections against Institutional Racism and Precarity

These themes have so far shown how participants described vaccination as a generally good thing but approached each vaccine decision as personal, contextual, and as filtered through their experiences as racialized refugees. In theme 3 (distrust of racially exclusive evidence), participants argued that clinical evidence did not derive from, address, and respond to their embodied histories, realities, and needs; in this sixth theme, participants argue more forcefully that the very institutions advising them to vaccinate—public health, medicine, school—were the same institutions in which they experienced discrimination and exclusion. Participants described their vaccine dissent as an active, protective disengagement from the institutions perpetuating their oppression.

Across interviews, mothers frequently referenced historical, contemporary, and personal experiences of medical racism as foundational to their hesitations about vaccines. Three parents referenced the Tuskegee experiments as evidence that US medical practice was anchored in a racist past and could not be accepted at face value. One Somali American activist told me that everyone knew about Tuskegee; Tuskegee circulated through Somali networks of transnational communication and served as a shorthand that warned people to scrutinize medical recommendations (2/2/2018). Interviews demonstrated that circulating anxieties about the history of medical racism in the US were concretized as resettled Somalis began to interact with US healthcare. Among the 24 parents interviewed, 16 participants related experiences of medical discrimination, harm, neglect, or all three as confirming their worries that US healthcare was not a system that prioritized their well-being. Five participants told stories about their children being prescribed antibiotics and suffering side effects. All five participants also described a sense of abandonment when they sensed something was amiss and tried to secure medical help. One participant recalled bringing her five-year-old daughter into the emergency room when she was having ongoing stomach pain, only to be sent home; "There was no way to contact a doctor. They said she was fine. I had to pay them $200 to do nothing" (7/20/2018). Three participants referenced traumatic experiences with cesarean births. Of these three participants, one concluded, "Long story short, they just don't know how to take care of Somalis here" (12/5/2018). Nine participants explained that because they were on public health insurance, they expected to receive substandard care. One participant explained, "They already think we don't know anything. They see the hijab, they see four, five, six kids, and they think we are a drain. Add that," and she gestured to the insurance card, "they think they can't get anything from us, and we have no power to get better medicine" (3/23/2018). These statements attest to a felt truth, what sociologist Arlie Hochschild (2020) has called a "deep story." This felt truth was that Somali Americans did not matter in medical institutions in the same ways that white, US-born people mattered.

Healthcare was not the only institution in which Somali refugees experienced discrimination; as a result, Somali American parents sometimes situated vaccine refusal as a form of protective withdrawal from the intersecting harms they faced in institutions writ large. Here, Farhiyo's homespun etiology of autism is instructive. Farhiyo's argument captures her inherently suspicious stance[5] against powerful and expert institutions. Farhiyo had made different vaccination decisions for each of her three children. She related that Somali American children were uniquely at risk of developing more disabling forms of autism, and that vaccination played a role in this risk. Farhiyo offered the following reasons for her autism worries:

---

5. Refer to Charles (2018, 2022) for a theorization of suspicion.

There are three reasons: immunizations, climate, food. Do you believe that people grow where they are supposed to? You take everyone, all of us Somali people, who are used to a climate, a geography, and then you move us here, where there's wind, snow, and hail. Our bodies must adjust, and it's not easy, it's not where we're used to and where we've grown to be.

In Somalia, everything we eat is fresh. We don't have refrigerators. You're ready to make dinner? You go out to the market, you get your food, you get your meat, which was killed that morning. We didn't have bread that you could keep for two weeks. Here, there's only a dollar store with canned food.

There's also where we live. We're living in places where people have never lived before. And we're low-income, so they crowd us next to a mine or a factory or a plant, and there's voltage and toxins. Nobody has lived there before, and now there are all these Somalis crowded there. They're exposed to toxins every day, and mothers know it's making their kids sick, but there's nothing to do about it. Our bodies weren't meant for this place. And vaccination is the same thing. It works differently on our bodies—you put it all together, and it's too much for a body to handle. (3/19/2018)

Farhiyo's vaccine suspicion was fueled by her day-to-day experiences of community sickness, of being neglected by the institutions that were supposed to protect public interests. Farhiyo described living in a place where she could not access healthy food, safe housing, or clean air. Accordingly, Farhiyo defined autism as an illness caused by a confluence of environmental factors, including vaccination as well as the unknown health consequences of displacement, diet, stress, environmental pollutants, and environmental racism. Indeed, in the US, race is the most consistent predictor of toxic-waste exposure, and, tellingly, undervaccination (Taylor, 2014). Farhiyo described vaccination as one more foreign intervention entering her children's displaced and structurally vulnerable bodies: "We all see it: there's new things entering our bodies, and our kids are sick" (3/19/2018). These experiences made it illogical to trust medical interventions endorsed by the same institutions that kept these structural inequities in place. "Daily life," Hausman reminds us, "provides a powerful set of experiences that frame alternative worldviews that may or may not align with the technocratic framing of data" (2019, p. 212). Daily life provided Farhiyo with ample evidence that her health was low on the list of public concern.

When participating parents felt that their children's health was, at once, uniquely imperiled by Western life and not valued by public institutions, parents described nonvaccination as protection. Participants did not have the power to protect their children from the health threats enumerated by

Farhiyo, including pollution, discrimination at school, unstable food access, subpar housing, and pervasive medical racism. But they could make decisions about vaccines. Vaccine refusals like Farhiyo's can be read as insistences that the structural problems that affect the health of Somali American children matter and as constrained acts of somatic protection.

Theme 7: Adaptive Protection When There's No Safety Net

Nonvaccination as protective care was especially necessary for participants who knew that they could not trust healthcare to help them should their children incur a vaccine injury, however rare. Somali parents' worries that routine vaccinations might prove uniquely risky for Somali American children were intensified when parents also realized how costly healthcare was. If a child was to have a bad reaction to a vaccine, who would help? At what cost? Dehka explained that she felt wary of accepting any kind of medical tool that might induce her to rely on more medical tools, as she had experienced US healthcare as impossibly expensive and difficult to access. Dehka explained the logic undergirding her nonvaccination:

> I believe that the vaccines protect against diseases, the measles vaccine protects kids from measles, the chickenpox vaccine protects them from chickenpox, but what will the side effects be? Most children, they do get better from measles, chickenpox, flu. But vaccine sicknesses, autism, other side effects, developmental disabilities, you're on your own, and no one knows what to do. No one helps you if a child reacts. (3/1/2018)

Dehka explained that she would rather take on a risk she felt personally equipped to understand and treat (measles, flu, chickenpox) than expose her family to risk that would make them dependent on medical expertise and intervention (vaccine injury). Dehka's statement could be read as a symptom of a wrong belief that the MMR vaccine can cause autism, but I argue that Dehka's statement is more a protective, logical recognition of and response to a costly and inaccessible healthcare system. Dehka knew that if her child were to have a vaccine injury, she would be on her own to navigate the potentially lifelong social, financial, and logistical fallouts. Thus, her statement is less an erroneous claim and more a strategy to avoid even the slimmest chance of incurring an injury that would necessitate further dependence on a bureaucratic, expensive, and individualistic healthcare system. Participants like Dehka learned that they could not rely on healthcare to protect their children, and so they practiced healthcare measures that allowed them the greatest possibility of control. Doing so meant turning away from expert systems and their tools. Vaccine refusal was one strategy among many for parents to care for their children, who were overexposed to health risks and under-resourced when it came to accessing medical knowledge and healthcare resources. In this reality, parents could only trust themselves.

Tracing Rhetorical Refusal's Arc through Vaccine Dissent

Somali participants' accounts of their outbreak and vaccination experiences bring a broader context of nonvaccination into focus. Their stories do not extol nonvaccination as the right decision, but they do allow for nonvaccination to speak, to buzz with rhetoricity and meaning, to point to other problems—beyond individual beliefs and vaccine decisions—that merit attention, resources, and redress. These stories make space for vaccine refusal to not just *refuse* vaccines but to *rhetorically refuse* compliance to institutions complicit in oppression. As discussed in this book's introduction, Smilges (2022) has urged rhetoricians to turn our scholarship "away from what people are saying to what they aren't, away from who is speaking to who is remaining silent, and away from speech entirely toward the ways silence has been signifying all along" (p. 9). Rhetorical, embodied vaccine refusals are signifying silences; they are activist optings-out, protective enclosures, and generative openings. Somali American parents' vaccine refusals coupled with parents' stories chart rhetorical refusal's situated arc: its exigence, usefulness, and generativity. Participating parents' rhetorical refusals grew from exigences of structural exclusion from the public good. Parents' rhetorical refusals protected children from structural racism, from underresearched refugee health concerns, and from ongoing precarity in resettlement—that is, from community sickness. Parents' refusals forged discursive space for new models of community health, clinical research, and clinical evidence. These are exigences, uses, and arcs of Somali American participants' vaccine refusals that I describe in the remainder of this chapter.

Refusal's Exigence:
Vaccine Dissent in Response to Exclusion from the Herd

The success of vaccination relies on herd immunity and community buy-in, or the willingness of each of us to take on a small risk, even a risk as small as a brief sting at the injection site, for the benefit of the population (Lawrence,

2020, pp. 110–115). However, Somali American participants told story after story of being excluded from the herd, the public of public health. Participants spoke to experiences of living in crowded apartment buildings alongside highways, cut off from grocery stores and green spaces. Participants spoke to experiences of having their children disciplined, surveilled, and unsupported at school. Participants described healthcare providers as dismissive of them, their questions, and their experiences, such as receiving multiple rounds of vaccination in migration. Participants described a dearth of reliable, affordable housing. These accretive experiences, even though most have nothing directly to do with vaccination, left participants with the lived knowledge that they, as members of a racialized immigrant population, were not included in the concept of the social good. Appeals to vaccinate as a means for protecting the public and upholding one's social responsibility therefore rang false. Claims about distributed risk and shared benefits clashed with participants' experiences of community sickness and its dismissal. Somali American participants' vaccine dissent is therefore a testament to what happens when the public of public health becomes glaringly inequitable. This fractured public of public health breaks down into a rich soil for nonvaccination.

Refusal's Usefulness: Protection from the Margins

Somali American participants, managing community sickness on their own, used vaccine dissent as an embodied form of protection. Participants disengaged from institutions bound up in their marginalization and enacted rhetorical refusal as a protective enclosure. Unable to trust that the public protected by public health policy included them, Somali American parents relied on their own knowledge and on self-administered care to cultivate their children's health. By refusing vaccines, Somali American parents described protecting their children against racist and discriminatory healthcare interactions. Parents described protecting their children from potential harms of trusting medical evidence grounded in the somatic experiences of white nonimmigrants. Parents described practicing healthcare in ways that afforded them the most control, in ways that reduced their chanced of being roped into a costly, uncaring healthcare system. Toward this goal of protection, participating parents described spreading out vaccines or waiting until children were older to administer vaccines. Somali American parents avoided not just vaccines but also antibiotics, sanitizers, processed foods, too much cold weather, new stressors, and pollutants. Selective nonvaccination was one protective health practice among many others that parents devised to protect children when they had few other means of control and protection available.

Refusal's Arc: What Is a Healthy Community?

Somali American parents' rhetorical vaccine refusals were also generative in that these refusals reimagined healthy communities beyond compliance, high vaccination rates, and control of disease. Typically, public health approaches identify a healthy community as, foundationally, one where there is high vaccination compliance and no disease outbreak. Lawrence (2020) has shown that this model of community health is grounded in the implicit recognition of eradication as the "material exigence" of vaccination, meaning that eradication is the primary driver and outcome of effective vaccine policy (pp. 49–59). Eradication, as a material exigence for vaccination policy, prioritizes getting everyone vaccinated, through whatever means necessary. Eradication can have the unintended effect of keeping disease elimination and individuals' personal vaccine decision-making in perpetual odds, as every decision to not vaccinate is coded as an obstruction to eradication rather than, say, an opportunity to rethink vaccination policy and public health goals or as a sign that current policies are not working (Lawrence, 2020, p. 64). Eradication, as a material exigence, endorses policies that keep vaccination rates high, such as tighter vaccine mandates, but forecloses public health efforts that are not explicitly tied to increasing vaccine compliance. Eradication, as the chief exigence for and goal of vaccination policy, leaves little rhetorical room to consider other avenues, beyond compliance and disease elimination, toward community health (Lawrence, 2020, pp. 72–74). Therefore, the resulting vaccine policy may increase vaccination rates but not necessarily public trust.

Interviewed Somali American mothers described a healthy community outside of the metric of eradication. Participants described a healthy community as one where there was widespread access to stable housing and healthy food. Healthcare was affordable. Sick people stayed home, rested, and were cared for on their own bodies' timelines. Refugees had healthcare that responded to their specific needs. A healthy community was one that responded to the causes of community sickness. When that kind of healthy community exists, vaccine compliance can follow. But before that kind of healthy community exists, all the energy put into vaccine compliance felt, to many participants, like a technical distraction from bigger health concerns. In chapter 1, Somali American participants used the term *community sickness* to expand understandings of disease causation to social, economic, and political factors and historical contexts. In this chapter, Somali American parents responded to the obscured exigence of community sickness with nonvaccination, a nonaction that signifies, that insists that vaccines are not normatively neutral, that unveils the ways that vaccines "function structurally and rhetorically as ways of avoiding addressing the systemic problems that cause outbreaks" (Lawrence, in Welhausen et al., 2015, p. 9), and that opens deliberative space to envision community health outside of or in addition to eradication. Somali American parents' rhetorical refusals were generative in that they forged discursive space for a more challenging but possibly more sustainable and collaborative model of community health.

Refusal's Arc: What If the Risk Is Real?

Somali American participants' rhetorical refusals were participatory in a second, novel way: Somali American participants refused clinical evidence drawn from the idea of a universal human body, and their dissent, in turn, arced toward clinical research responsive to experiential expertise. So far, my analysis of Somali American parents' vaccine refusals has sidestepped an important dimension of participants' arguments: parents expressed concerns about physical harms that vaccines might bring to Somali American children. Participants raised concerns about the interplays of abrupt dietary, environmental, and healthcare (including vaccination) changes. What happened when you ate exclusively fresh foods and then switched to preserved and refrigerated foods? What happened when you moved from an equatorial climate to a Northern, cold one? What about the health effects of living through civil war, famine, and forced migration? Participants expressed concerns about how healthcare providers treated them and whether racism, anti-immigrant sentiments, and Islamophobia impacted their health. Participants worried that multiple rounds of the same vaccine administered at different points of migration might harm their children. Participants worried that their children's bodies might be marked by migration and stress in ways that made them newly allergic to vaccines. Participants questioned how seriously they should take medical evidence that did not come from studies on displaced people. Again and again, there was the following concern: but you haven't tested this vaccine *on someone like me*.

In the health literacy frame, these concerns about vaccines are bundled and homogenized under the label of vaccine hesitancy. They are then labeled as incorrect. They are explained away as the misgivings of persons unversed in science. In humanistic and social science approaches, these concerns are often read as idioms for broader, complex social issues. Scholars have shown that what gets expressed as a concern about a specific vaccine might *really* be the expression of concerns about modernity (Hausman, 2017; Hausman, 2019), globalizing technocracies and their colonizing histories (Charles, 2022), the political economies in which vaccines are embedded (Leach and Fairhead, 2007), racism in medicine (Campeau, 2019), and the ways that scientific institutions have participated in historical social injustices (Goldenberg, 2021). In these studies, vaccine hesitancy isn't about the vaccine; hesitancy is a metacommentary about something bigger. But what if it is about the vaccine? What if these risks are worth looking into on their own accord?[6] To automatically read participants' vaccine anxieties as either signs of ignorance or as referents to something else, even if that something else is important, is to strip these concerns of their intention, detail, experiential evidence, and potential for offering empirical evidence, beyond the anecdote, synecdoche, or metaphor. Somali American parents' vaccine concerns, informed by embodied experience, have potential as "contributory expertise" (Collins and Evans, 2002), lived evidence that might nonetheless be scientifically valuable. Somali American parents' rhetorical vaccine refusals situate migration, racialization, and structural marginalization not just as experiences that might mark a population but as sites for contesting scientific knowledge and for forging new insights. In this longer, concluding section, I take seriously the question built into participants' dissent: What if the risk is real?

Somali American participants' embodied concerns are not without precedent. There is evidence that pharmaceuticals do not work in the same way for everyone and that disease mechanisms are not universal across all persons and populations. Much Western medical knowledge comes from studies of how diseases, injuries, and therapeutic responses manifest in white, male bodies (Clayton and Collins, 2014; Oh et al., 2015). In 1993, the National Institutes of Health (NIH) instituted the Revitalization Act, which required inclusion of both women and minorities in NIH clinical research and disclosure of research participant demographics; since then, NIH-funded studies have included large proportions of women and racial and ethnic minorities by design and have made clinically relevant scientific contributions, most often by identifying sex-specific differences in symptoms, pathologies, and treatment responses (Oh et al., 2015; Canto et al., 2007; Hoffman and Tarzian, 2001). But studies conducted prior to 1993 still provide much of the evidence used to inform clinical practices. Evidence also shows that race and ethnicity can predict differential bodily responses to pharmaceuticals. Race is not a biological characteristic but rather "a social construct rooted in cultural identity and shaped by historic and current events, which influence an individual's behavior and place of residence" (Oh et al., 2015), but because genetic differences can affect clinical presentation and therapeutic responses and because

---

6. Thank you to reader 1 for posing this question and providing the infrastructure for this argument.

racial categories have been shown to correlate with genetic differences, race and ethnicity can stand as useful proxies for genetic variations. For these reasons, intentional racial diversity in clinical trials has led to clinically significant findings (Wu et al., 2015). To give one example, the blood thinner clopidogrel (Plavix) was discovered not to work in 75% of Pacific Islanders, those whose bodies do not produce the enzyme required to activate the drug. The drug also bears for Pacific Islanders a heightened risk of heart attack and stroke (Wu et al., 2015). Plavix was approved by the FDA in 1997, and this warning for Pacific Islanders and people of East Asian descent was not added until 2010. The black-box warning was added because of a lawsuit informed by the advocacy by Hawaiian people taking Plavix as prescribed, reporting no benefits, and suffering heart attacks (Wu et al., 2015). Put differently, everyday peoples' anecdotal evidence and subsequential advocacy led to the reexamination of this pharmaceutical and its proven safety and effectiveness. Asked in an interview about race-based disparities in responses to asthma medications, epidemiologist Sam S. Oh responded, "You begin to wonder, 'Well, why is this the case?' And part of that reason might be because our biomedical studies in the past have not recruited as heavily in those populations [African Americans and Hispanic Americans]" (as qtd. in Bichell, 2015). Oh was being interviewed about his 2015 study that found there is not enough clinical data to confidently make health recommendations to people from nondominant racial and ethnic groups.

Genetic variations from clinical findings hold true for some vaccine responses, too. There is an increased disease burden for Hib among Native American children, and thus there are personalized vaccine recommendations that Native American children receive additional or preferential delivery of Hib vaccinations (Hammitt, 2019). As well, there was a genetic link between the 2009–2010 flu vaccine Pandemrix and increased risk for narcolepsy in Sweden (Partinen et al., 2012; Heier et al., 2013; Weibel et al., 2018; CDC, 2020). Researchers found that the Pandemrix vaccine potentially triggered antibodies that bind to the receptor in brain cells that helps regulate sleepiness; Pandemrix likely triggered an autoimmune reaction that led to narcolepsy in a small group of people who were genetically at risk (Vogel, 2015; Hallberg et al., 2019). In other words, a small population, united by genetic similarities, had a negative reaction to a vaccine that was harmless to most of its recipients. This explanation mirrors Somali American parents' concerns that a vaccine that worked for most people might still affect Somali diaspora children differently.

Citizen-led health movements, too, have yielded insights about health and disease. In citizen-science undertakings, people have contested science with evidence built from their embodied knowledge (Epstein, 1996; Brown and

Mikkelson, 1998; Brown, 2007; Alaimo, 2010). Sociologists Phil Brown and Edwin J. Mikkelson (1998) followed a group of residents of Woburn, Massachusetts, who suspected that contaminated well water was causing a childhood leukemia cluster in their town. Initially, the residents failed to convince anyone in power to take them seriously, but they translated their embodied experiences and related "local epidemiologies" into scientific-enough terms, gained the attention and collaboration of scientists, and sued the two seemingly untouchable corporations that were contaminating their water source. In later work, Brown and collaborators have documented similarly impactful—and always initially doubted—citizen science projects related to environmental causes of breast cancer (McCormick et al., 2004; Brown, 2007), asthma (Brown et al., 2004; Brown, 2007), Gulf War syndrome (Zavestoski et al., 2004; Brown, 2007), and per- and polyfluoroalkyl substances (PFAS) contamination (Ohayon et al., 2023).

With hindsight on our side, it is easier to categorize citizen-science movements as either brave and pioneering or as misguided or malevolent, but during a movement, these distinctions are not so clear. Medical anthropologist Danya Glabau (2022) has categorized the health activism championed by "mother's movements" into two such categories. There is the antiscience antivaccination movement, which Glabau uses as an example of the misguided citizen-science project. By contrast, there are mother-activists who do "not seek to replace the epistemic authority of technoscientific expertise but to improve it—what might be seen as enacting a 'feminist science'" (p. 21). These activists try to "answer situated questions that are specific to children and women and their everyday lives" (p. 21). In this second category, Glabau includes the "radiation brain mom" activists in Japan who organized in response to environmental contamination after the Fukushima nuclear disaster (Kimura, 2016). These two categories—mother-led movements that seek to supplant science versus those that advance science—make sense when attached to clear, post hoc examples. But it's not always clear which citizen-led movements are onto something or not. And, as I argued in the beginning of this chapter, the staple caricature of the deluded, too-educated-for-her-own-good antivax mom rhetorically disables arguments that mothers might raise about vaccines. One important function of rhetorical refusal is to position nonscientific claims as potentially useful, informed not by medical expertise but expertise nonetheless. Put simply, rhetorical refusals can work in an epistemic way to flag potentially real health problems. Are Somali mothers' vaccine concerns without substance, or might they be attempts to "answer situated questions that are specific to children and women and their everyday lives" (Glabau, 2022, p. 21)? The literacy, culture, and trust frames of medical dissent, as well as the wrong-belief frame of vaccine controversy, only allow for consideration of vaccine hesitancy as wrong and fixable; in these frames, even considering the latter question is a move against science and toward the dangerous waters of antivaccination. Rhetorical refusal, however, allows listeners to consider the latter option without compromising their confidence in vaccination and science.

As rhetorical refusals, parents' noncompliant vaccinations raise concerns with the applicability of evidence drawn from clinical trials and call for change in how medical evidence is produced. When Somali American parents' rhetorical vaccine refusals are contextualized in social-scientific research about the clinical trial industry, however, it becomes clear that the solution is not to recruit study participants from different racial backgrounds and to conduct more racially diverse clinical trials. Sociologist Stephen Epstein (2007) has shown how policy to diversify clinical trials has done more to produce new problems than to correct a lack of race and gender representation in clinical trials. Policy to diversify clinical trials has led research teams, under pressure to qualify for funding and produce results fast, to resort to bean-counting retrofits rather than meaningful inclusion of diverse participants. As a result, studies are designed to over-recruit marginalized participants, sometimes in predatory ways; check diversity boxes; and ask research questions that reify biological markers of difference. The question, as Epstein puts it, "is not whether to study race, but how to study it"—and mandating diverse representation in clinical trials is not the way forward (p. 231).

Further to this point, clinical trials in the US *have* become more diverse—phase 1 clinical trial participants are now mostly young Black and Hispanic men—but this representation has not led to improved health outcomes. Social scientist Jill A. Fisher's ethnographic study of phase 1 clinical trials (2020) depicts how trials exploit social inequality and how social inequalities warp clinical findings. The economic pressure that often motivates people to enroll in trials also motivates participants to bend study protocols (skipping "wash-out" periods, participating serially in studies) and to mold their bodies into ideal laboratory specimen, the kinds of bodies that will pass screenings and earn study stipends, but also the kinds of bodies that have little similarity to the bodies of non–trial participants. Fisher concluded her ethnographic research with a grave warning for public health:

> Phase I clinical trials come with a host of intrinsic and extrinsic validity problems that raise public health concerns. [. . .] The safety profile of FDA-approved drugs remains largely unknown. Despite the appearance that FDA-approved drugs have been proven safe, this perception is just a myth propagated by the pharmaceutical industry and supported by the regulatory system. (p. 255)

Fisher's work lends unexpected credence to Somali American parents' concerns that the evidence produced by clinical trials may not be valid for them. Epstein's and Fisher's scholarship contends that the pharmaceutical industry exploits social inequality to fill their clinical trials. This is the same social inequality that Somali American participants referred to as contributing to community sickness and which has compelled parents' distrust in vaccines and public health expertise. Fisher's conclusions suggest that the same sources of community sickness that sparked Somali American mothers' distrust in pharmaceutical products also dilute clinical evidence. Somali American parents' rhetorical vaccine refusals can contribute to calls to reform clinical trials.

To conclude, rhetorical refusals work not just in a symbolic way but in an epistemic way. Rhetorical refusals can raise real health concerns and inform scientific progress. Somali American vaccine dissent is not only rhetorically powerful but also potentially clinically relevant. Rhetorical refusals offer "contributory expertise" (Collins and Evans, 2002) or embodied "counter-knowledge" (Goldenberg, 2021) that might work in an epistemic way to flag real health problems. This epistemic potential of vaccine refusal has rarely been studied, perhaps because acknowledging that vaccine refusal might have an epistemic function seems to tread too closely to vaccine refusal itself. Instead, humanists invested in the work of really understanding—and not just quickly correcting—vaccine hesitancy have largely described vaccine hesitancy as a synecdoche for a larger, systemic, harder-to-put-into-words concerns. *Rhetorical refusal,* as a rhetorical concept, builds on such work but also insists on listening to participants' claims that vaccines might bear real health risks for them. Listening to rhetorical refusal involves taking these embodied experiences seriously, even if they do not align with the existing scientific evidence. Embodied rhetorical refusals can therefore advance meaningful critique of the production of scientific knowledge and can help develop scientific knowledge and guide its applications. Embodied rhetorical refusals are useful to raise critiques about how Western medicine works as a system, how specific medicines work on specific bodies, and how medicine can respond to the contextualized needs of marginalized groups.

Conclusion

In this chapter, I have shown how the published news and public health accounts of the 2017 Minnesota measles outbreak offered a consistent but incomplete outbreak story. These discourses situated Somali parents as the passive grounds on which battles between antivaccination groups and public health institutions were fought. Somali parents were characterized by a lack of scientific knowledge that rendered them vulnerable to others' arguments and interests. Whichever group, antivaxxers or public health, could get to Somali people first and in the most engaging ways would win. This narrative allowed no rhetorical space for Somali Americans to have informed views about vaccines, medicine, and health. Somali persons were characterized as scientifically uninformed, easily led astray. Their words could offer only misappropriations of scientific knowledge.

Somali American parents' stories shattered this framing. Interviewed parents drew from experiential, communal, and medical knowledges and made situational vaccine decisions to protect their children as they engaged with unjust systems. Participants' embodied vaccine refusals were generative acts of participation that reimagined healthy communities and clinical research. Following participants' refusals leads away from the question of how vaccination communication can be more persuasive and toward questioning what types of knowledge, forms of collaboration, and models of community health get erased in a singular focus on increasing vaccination compliance. In participants' outbreak stories, vaccine refusal and vaccine compliance do not exist in strict opposition. Rather, participants' stories enact vaccine refusal as a generative stance that can offer constructive ways of responding to racialized, gendered, historical, and affective politics of care. Vaccine refusals are forms of on-the-ground protection that people take up to care for themselves, their families, and their communities in structurally unjust worlds. Rhetorical vaccine refusals are embodied moves that insist on more just and healthy communities and more just research practices that prioritize public health. Vaccine refusals have the power to surface critiques that might have medical value to understanding how vaccines and other biotechnologies work, specifically for populations underrepresented in medical research.

The following chapters expand beyond vaccine refusal to other, less buzzy but important sites of refusal. These sites—refusing disability services through mistakes, silences, and failures and refusing medical therapies through alternative care—offer a fuller account of how rhetorical refusal works. The next chapter engages refusals of disability social services. These refusals build on this chapter's analysis about healthy communities while also mapping how rhetorical refusals work in systems of bureaucratic documentation. To do so, the next chapter engages less-studied spaces of healthcare, such as the social services office, the disability-specific support group, or the caseworker's house visit.

CHAPTER 3

Writing to the State

Mistakes and Silences as Rhetorical Refusal

In September 2017, as the measles outbreak was fading from local and national press, eight people gathered in a conference room in Midnimo. There were three members of Midnimo leadership, two Midnimo community health workers, two social-service staff, and myself, present as an observer. The group had gathered to hash out the terms of an autism support grant designed to serve Somali American families. The measles outbreak had made Somali American concerns about autism urgent, such that state and city agencies were freshly focused on providing services and outreach to their Somali residents (Midnimo's health literacy course, described in chapter 1, was supported by this wave of funding). In the months following the outbreak, state agencies awarded grants to expand autism services for Somali Americans. One grant recipient, Wingham County, used funding to build a bridge grant program for Somali American families. These grants, called the Wingham County Autism Grants (WCAG), were designed to provide easy-to-access, stop-gap funding to qualifying families; the grant would provide recipients with immediate funds while county staff worked with families to secure long-term services. The WCAG grant administrators sought to partner with Somali organizations, including Midnimo, to reach Somali families.

Malyun, Midnimo's executive director, wavered about whether to partner with Wingham County social services. Malyun worried that the grant would result in more of the same for her overpromised and underdelivered Somali clients. "I've done so many trainings for these human services departments," Malyun explained. "These are our cultural norms, blah blah. This is why some of us shake hands and some of us don't [. . .] and here are a few Somali words! They love learning Somali words. And then they're done. Moms come to me, say they've been waiting for years for a waiver, or they say their PCA is abusing a kid but they're afraid to report. No one hears these stories" (1/2/2018).

Ultimately, Malyun, on behalf of Midnimo, agreed to the WCAG partnership. In the partnership, Wingham County funded Midnimo to administer educational autism workshops and help participants write WCAG proposals. On their end, Midnimo recruited Somali parents to apply for the WCAG and attended county service-provider resource fairs. The partnership was in place. Midnimo gathered 26 mothers to participate in the WCAG program. The timeline was short, so the program moved fast. We were soon explaining the application process to 26 Somali American mothers in Midnimo's conference room. We were scanning handwritten applications to the county and driving updated diagnostic materials to the county offices; we were attending trainings, updating parents on the status of their applications, recruiting new families, and calling the county with a backlog of questions. But when the pace slowed, and we had time to check our numbers, the realization was inescapable: Malyun had been right. The grant was not working. When the program was over, only six of the original 26 Somali American families recruited received any funding. Midnimo cut off talks with the county team about future collaborations.

What had gone wrong? This chapter maps how the grant program fractured. The first part of the chapter contextualizes public assistance as a situated, historicized concept within the Somali diaspora. American social services held great allure for many Somali newcomers, but, in use, these services proved culturally abrasive and limited by neoliberal policies. After contextualizing state aid, the chapter zooms in on the documents that Somali American parents encountered when they began the WCAG application. Beginning with paperwork might appear a boring way to begin this story, but these documents are consequential in large part because of their veneer of dull necessity. These documents brought together parents, community health workers, and social service staff, and they coordinated how parents presented their children to the state and how the state evaluated family deservingness and endorsed or denied types of care.

During the WCAG application writing and reporting processes, which happened at this documentation interface, there occurred four junctures at which parent applicants failed to meet the WCAG requirements and departed from the program. These junctures were as follows: diagnosis, when parent applicants provided a medical diagnosis of autism; disclosure, when parents supplied personal family and health information and had county assessors visit their home to verify written claims; fundable plans, when parents proposed the types of care or services for which they sought funding; and caregiving relationships, when parents appointed and justified caregivers and their pay. These junctures were marked by mistakes, incorrect documentation, blank forms, unsubmitted applications, and departures from the grant program. At these junctures, parents provided medical documentation of diagnoses that were not autism; parents missed home visits; parents requested unfundable supports like rent aid or a trip to Somalia; parents submitted incomplete caregiving time sheets. On one hand, these actions could be read as symptoms of low health and bureaucratic literacies. They might be read as fixable mistakes, as opportunities to provide more training to Somali Americans about state processes, about what counts as medical care and what does not count. But I read these junctures as rhetorical refusals replete with meaning and disruptive resonance. Twenty Somali applicants abandoned the WCAG program not because they could not complete the applications but because they would not. They refused. Within the institutional documents themselves, there was little space to voice dissent or alternate views, except through mistakes, blank answers, and departures. This chapter addresses how rhetorical refusals signify within such rigid, one-way, bureaucratic writing situations. Rhetorical refusal is a concept useful to read institutional writing situations "against the grain" (Hartman, 2007) and follow the half-told stories and signifying silences (Smilges, 2022) folded into wrong answers, blank spaces, and missing forms toward what could be. The ways that Somali parent-authors refused to engage correctly with these documents tell important stories and add depth to the concept of rhetorical refusal, particularly in how rhetorical refusal works in top-down processes and how these rhetorical refusals interrupt neutralized ableist logics.

Public Assistance: Diaspora Visions and Resettled Realities

When Somali parents arrived at Midnimo to complete their WCAG applications, many came with preexisting relationships to and perceptions of public services and state aid. Often, perceptions were shaped by shared imaginaries of public services that circulated in refugee camps and diaspora communities, as well as firsthand experiences with government aid. Sociologist Cawo Abdi's (2015b) multisite ethnographic study of Somali diaspora depicts how public assistance emerged as an organizing principle and a sustaining imaginary for many Somali refugees. Stories of government aid circulated in Somalia, refugee camps, and common midmigration landing spots like Kenya and the United Arab Emirates (pp. 170–179); these stories tended to convey that the United States was the best place for resettlement because there were social supports for refugees. In the US, Somali immigrants imagined, they would be supported with government aid to get a job, provide for their families, and send meaningful remittances to kin (Horst, 2006; Abdi, 2015, pp. 172–175; Somalis in Minnesota Oral History Project, 2016).

For those who resettled in the US, the reality of government aid was more complicated and disillusioning. Most Somali refugees arrived in the US directly from refugee camps, some came through family reunification, and a much smaller number came through secondary migration from Europe or Canada (Berns-McGown, 1999; Abdi, 2015b). Escaping war and famine, many Somali refugees arrived in the US with no money or capital. US refugee resettlement assistance—made up of federal, state, and independent religious and civic organizations—therefore played a large role in the lives of newly arrived Somalis. When Somali refugees landed at American ports, they were received by volunteer agencies, which, in collaboration with federal and state resettlement agencies, transported refugees to allocated housing and guided newcomers through employment steps, housing referrals, school enrollments, and the procurement of clothing, food, and necessities. From there, Somalis, like other newly arrived refugees, usually engaged with welfare systems such as the Minnesota Family Investment Program.

Public assistance, however, worked in troubling ways for many Somali newcomers. Welfare rules disrupted stability-providing gender roles and religious and cultural norms at an already stressful time for families (Abdi, 2014). For example, in two-parent families, welfare applications were filed in the mother's name; this meant that the mother was listed as the "head of household," a role that in Somali culture belonged to the father. At a time when few Somali men could find work reliable and remunerative enough to support their families, this "head of household" designation was a hard pill to swallow. It meant that men had to step aside while checks arrived in their wives' names, and families had to readjust around or be pulled apart by these new gender roles (Abdi, 2014). Further, welfare funding was rarely sufficient to live on while families and individuals figured out their footing (Abdi, 2015b). Welfare's focus on getting a job quickly did long-term disservice to newcomers. Many Somali refugees were mothers arriving with multiple children, little formal education or transferable skills, and no English language literacy; still, they were funneled into welfare systems that prioritized getting a job as fast as possible, and so Somali refugees received little support to learn English, pursue education, or develop job-ready skills. They were jettisoned into whatever positions were available to them, which tended to be janitorial work and care-chain work for women and factory work for men, work that was precarious, low-paid, and did not support them to build skills (Abdi, 2015b; Kleist and Thorsen, 2016). These opposed demands of public assistance—to find a job as quickly as possible, but with the only jobs available paying unlivable wages— kept many Somalis locked in a poverty and welfare cycle. Government welfare agencies did not exist in Somalia, and in the US, Somali adults found their relationship to the state written into one of faceless dependence. It was within this system of heralded but ensnaring state support that autism social services emerged. Autism services brought their own challenges for Somali American families, whose needs these services were not at all designed to meet.

Autism Services: The Legacy of White Mothers' Activism

In the US, autism advocacy has historically been led by white, affluent mothers (Silverman, 2012; Decoteau, 2021). As a result, the structure of autism service provision has answered to the needs of white, affluent families. The pioneering activism led by white mothers in the mid-twentieth century led to broader coverage of autism services but also bore long-term exclusionary effects, including racializing autism as a white disorder and excluding from access to public services people of color, poor people, and people with higher service needs. In the 1980s, autism advocates, largely white mothers acting on behalf of their autistic children, argued that autism was a "looming epidemic," one that threatened to grow if the government did not intervene (Decoteau, 2021, p. 67). White mothers in the late twentieth century were in a similar rhetorical and epistemic position as Somali American parents were in the early twenty-first century: White activist mothers argued that autism cases were rising among their children, that no one understood why, and that something had to be done; in response, medical researchers and policymakers suggested that autism's increasing prevalence might not reflect an increase in autism so much as changes in autism detection and diagnosis procedures (Eyal et al., 2010; Orsini and Smith, 2010). This conflict mirrors the one that Somali American parents were in before the 2017 measles outbreak; Somali American parents argued that their children were part of poorly understood autism clusters, and experts offered other explanations: for example, maybe diagnostic methods were getting more equitable. White mother–led autism movements in the 1980s and 1990s, though, were successful in achieving the results activists desired. The "looming epidemic" argument—greased by its advocates' proximity to power—worked. This argument compelled the government to provide autism services at the same time as public services were elsewhere being scaled back under austerity measures to reduce costs in healthcare, education, and disability services. What resulted was the implementation of crisis-driven policies that focused on providing children with behavioral therapies before they reached the age of five, an age marked as a crucial "window of opportunity" in terms of childhood development and welfare savings for the state (Decoteau, 2021, p. 68).

Autism screenings and services had to be funded by a specific government entity, and so behavioral therapies were assigned to the jurisdiction of the healthcare system and were paid for by Medicaid waivers or insurance (Decoteau, 2021, pp. 67–70); this assignation shaped how behavioral therapies were delivered and measured. Broadly, to come under the purview of health insurance systems, behavioral therapies had to be supported by evidence from randomized control clinical trials, had to be delivered in standardized ways by accredited professionals, and had to be monitored by regulatory bodies. Advocacy groups led by white mothers again led the way; these groups fought for funding for randomized control trials of applied behavioral analysis therapy, and, in 1999, the US Surgeon General approved applied behavioral analysis therapy as sufficiently evidence-based. Insurance companies and state agencies were now responsible for covering the cost of newly legitimized applied behavioral analysis therapy (Decoteau, 2021, p. 73). Bureaucratic state task forces arose to discern eligibility and to oversee administration of applied behavioral analysis therapy (Silverman, 2012, pp. 98–100). These structures continue to affect who secures autism supports. Not only was applied behavioral analysis therapy itself reconfigured to fit into clinical and health insurance categories, but the prevailing path for securing services prioritized the needs, literacies, and norms of white parents, often at the expense of others. The advocacy of white mothers on behalf of their children institutionalized and made publicly accessible therapies and autism-specific resources, but these outcomes helped white, affluent families without lifting others up with them. Poor and immigrant households have languished at the bottom of long waitlists, and Somali Americans have been no exception. Decoteau quoted Adar, a Somali mother and autism advocate, as explaining,

> If you have money, if you can afford to pay [for] everything like the diet, you can hire someone who works [with] the child. . . . At home, you have someone who is cooking, cleaning, that sort of thing. . . . [Then] mom is not actually overwhelmed, you can cope with that. . . . You have a child with autism,

> but you don't feel the stress, the financial stress, other stress that are coming on.... *And those are the people that are advocating for autism.* .... Wherever I go, I meet them. And they will shut me up, because... they are connected with politicians. They have connections with big companies. (2021, p. 91)

Medical autism services are technically available to anyone, but the protracted processes that parents must navigate exclude many people from services. As one Somali parent explained to Decoteau, "Nobody has ABA. Maybe the white people [laughter], they know things" (2021, p. 79). "Autism advocacy," Decoteau synthesized, "is shaped by the privileged and ignores the needs of the marginalized" (2021, p. 91).

The WCAG remains informed by this history of autism services, even as the WCAG administrators have tried to break out of historical patterns. The WCAG program began with the acknowledgment that social services were failing Somali American families, and this grant was therefore developed for them specifically. In the sections that follow, I argue that participating Somali parents' rhetorical refusals rejected not just the WCAG but long-standing foundations of autism services, mainly the premises that autism is an individual disability appropriately treated through medical therapies, that autistic children should be encouraged to progress toward an implicit model of a normal child, and that forms of care must be siloed within state agencies. Somali parents' rhetorical refusals therefore unsettle the norms that white mother–led autism advocacy had established as neutral and necessary. Before moving into actual rhetorical refusals, I look at the WCAG application itself, as it was within this three-page document that Somali mothers, social-service staff, county assessors, and Midnimo health workers were all brought into each other's orbits; it was within these three pages that parents articulated their rhetorical refusals.

The Paperwork: Outreach Materials, the Grant Application, and a Consumer-Directed Model of Care

Wingham County and Midnimo described the WCAG as a person-centered grant designed to meet the underserved needs of Somali American families. To be person-centered, the WCAG was designed to support the applicant's vision of what their family needed. In one of the initial emails describing the WCAG program, the county summarized the program's goal: "Modeled after self-directed programs, the grant team created a simple grant application form that asks individuals and families to define what supports would work best for them" (9/31/2018). WCAG administrator Jenn outlined this new model of person-centered or consumer-directed[1] disability funding to Midnimo parents with a two-column chart. The first column, labeled "traditional," illustrated an older, phasing-out model of services in which decisions were made by a case manager. This column included the following items:

- no paid spouse or parent option
- provider sets the rate
- provider writes the plan
- provider trains staff [. . .]
- provider hires staff
- provider helps develop health and safety plan
- provider only uses licensed services
- county approves plan. (WCAG workshop, 9/31/2018)

The second column, labeled "consumer-directed," described a new model wherein applicants made choices about their care, including who provided their care. This column featured the following list:

- paid parent or spouse
- person sets rate, writes plan, trains and hires staff, develops health and safety plan
- still: county approves plan. (WCAG workshop, 9/31/2018)

In a consumer-directed model of care, the applicant was not matched up with a state-funded personal care assistant (PCA); funds that would traditionally pay a PCA could be used to pay a person of the client's choosing, usually a family member. The client then participated in writing their care plan and goals, tasks that were formerly relegated to a state-appointed care team. "By person-centered," Jenn explained about the WCAG, "we mean it's not about what we think your child needs, it's about what you know your child needs. You're the parent. You're the expert" (2/22/2018).

After describing consumer-directed services, Jenn distributed the WCAG applications. The entire application was three sheets of paper stapled together. The WCAG's introduction explained that the purpose of the WCAG was to "meet individual needs" and "fill gaps in current services." The grant was designated to provide for "caregiver relief and community integration and provides flexibility for individuals and families to determine how best to meet

---

1. The county used the terms *person-centered* and *consumer-directed* interchangeably.

those needs for their situation." Next, the introduction provided the following list of fundable services:

- Licensed or non-licensed respite services
- Community engagement activities, such as adaptive recreation, social clubs, etc.
- Services or items to support community integration and valued social roles, such as behavioral support staff or a communication device.

"Respite services" were defined below as self-care practices for parents, while the second two options were focused on resources for the child.

Next, the introduction overviewed the grant procedure. The "individual, family, certified assessor, case manager or community member" would "identify unmet needs and appeal to the WCAG grant to meet these needs for 3–12 months." Jenn explained that during this time, the applicant should be working with social-service staff to prepare their applications for longer-term supports such as disability waivers.

After the introduction, there was a chart that requested the following identifying information: name, address, phone number, social security number, race, email, and case manager's name and email address. The grant specified two criteria for eligibility:

- Must have a diagnosis of autism spectrum disorder or related condition (please attach supporting documentation to application)
- Must reside in Wingham County.

Next, a series of short answer questions asked for the following information:

- Diagnosis,
- How disability disrupts family life,
- Services currently or previously used,
- Additional stresses for the family, such as single parent, family size, loss of job, other family members with disabilities, low income,
- Any informal supports used.

The final section asked applicants to identify and justify the services requested by answering the following three questions:

- Description of funding requested. How will funding be used?
- How is it related to disability?
- Sustainability of request.

The last item in the application asked for an applicant's budget and specified that the grants could fund proposals of up to $3,000. The application closed with a line requesting the applicant's signature. The WCAG application was short, but, as the next section explains, this slim packet engendered conflict, double binds, and rhetorical refusal.

Rhetorical Refusals through Mistakes, Silences, and Departures

Sitting before the WCAG application, the applicant was instructed to answer the questions, select from preidentified choices, supply requested information, and present appropriate evidence. Doing so meant that the parent, now applicant, mapped her child along the county's coordinates, told her child's story as filtered through the document's categories, made requests on behalf of the child in ways legible to the state, and then waited to see if the application would return resources. But some applicants did not follow these rules. Some Somali applicants composed rhetorical refusals—silences, wrong answers, incomplete answers, missed appointments. Such rhetorical refusals, made at the application interface, demonstrate how constrained rhetors communicate dissent and alternative visions in bureaucratic, top-down processes and documentation. The following four sites of rhetorical refusal map how parents communicated refusal in these rigid writing situations and depict how parents' rhetorical refusals unsettle normative conceptions of care, disability, parenting, and state aid.

Refusal 1: Diagnosis (8 Participants)

The first site of rhetorical refusal occurred when the WCAG necessitated that parents prove their eligibility by supplying medical documentation of a child's autism diagnosis. Much to the grant administrators' expressed surprise, few of Midnimo's recruited participants had anticipated this requirement, and many parents in attendance were there for children who did not have autism. One might think, well, of course, individuals without an autism diagnosis cannot get services set aside for individuals with autism. But there's more to it. Somali American parents' lack of diagnostic documentation speaks to the ways that medical diagnoses can fragment biosocial communities built on shared experiences of caregiving. Diagnoses can cut people off from previous social groups, grounded in shared experiences of illness and difference, and usher individuals into private patient-provider relationships and individualized caregiving. As a rhetorical refusal, an unsupplied medical diagnosis documentation rejects the requisite medicalization of disability and care.

Khadija's story exemplifies this rhetorical refusal. Khadija's story depicts how medical diagnoses can alienate applicants from not only the WCAG but also from social services and informal networks of care. At the first Midnimo-hosted WCAG workshop, I sat with Khadija, a Somali American mother who arrived to apply for the WCAG, and Molly, a Midnimo community health worker. Molly and Khadija moved quickly through the first questions on the WCAG; Khadija handed her state ID to Molly, who copied the requested information. The pair paused at the next section, "Eligibility," the first bullet point of which read, "Must have a diagnosis of autism spectrum disorder or related condition." Molly read the request aloud.

Khadija said, "They don't have autism."

"OK," Molly said. "That's OK, they take related conditions. Do your children have a diagnosis?"

Khadija explained that her son and daughter had a skin problem in which the slightest touch could cause bleeding. "They need to be wrapped in cold cloth to sleep at night," she said. "And they wake up screaming, even then, because the cloth cools and hardens and hurts their skin. I'm up all night, changing their sheets. They are always bleeding, and they get fevers."

Molly transcribed everything. "Is there anything," she asked, "like, do they have any trouble communicating?"

"They don't have friends," Khadija answered. "They're bullied."

"But they can speak?"

"Yes."

"I'm just," Molly explained, "I'm just looking for similarities between this condition and autism, looking for ways to categorize this as a related condition."

"They must have autism?" Khadija asked.

"Well, no, not 100% of the time, but it helps if we can say the condition is related, like if they have sensory troubles or communication troubles."

"I thought—[my friend] told me to come to Midnimo because they would help parents with sick kids, that there was money."

Molly assured Khadija that Midnimo would help her no matter what (1/22/2018). It was not until the parents had all gone home and Midnimo staff were photocopying the handwritten grant applications that we realized that Khadija was in the majority. Few mothers had arrived with an autism diagnosis in hand. Mothers had arrived on behalf of children with far-ranging diagnoses, including microcephaly, multiple sclerosis, ADHD, a heart problem, a gunshot injury, and an undiagnosed history of seizures. Twelve mothers arrived on behalf of children who had been diagnosed at school as having a developmental delay, but the developmental delay had not been confirmed as autism or examined by a physician. Out of the 26 mothers present, three had medical documentation in hand to verify an autism diagnosis. Including those three, 12 of the 26 mothers said that they were here for a child who had autism. Fourteen mothers arrived for reasons other than autism or were unclear about their child's diagnosis.

Over the next several weeks, parents brought to Midnimo medical documentation, and community health workers were dispatched to participants' homes to collect documentation. These exchanges often involved several attempts. Some parents brought in hospital discharge instructions describing unrelated injuries and events. Some parents brought in physicians' business cards and asked Midnimo staff to call the clinic and request records. Khadija brought a plastic grocery bag filled with medical documents. Molly sorted through the documents, selected materials, and submitted Khadija's application with the following explanation, written by Molly:

> **What is the applicant's diagnosis or disability?** Khadija's children have a severe skin condition called epidermolysis bullosa, in which their skin falls off and bleeds and their hair falls out. They must be very careful because even just rubbing against a hard surface can make them bleed for a long time. They frequently get fevers and have trouble sleeping because their skin is itching and burning. The caretaker burden here is related to that of autism because Khadija's children need near-constant supervision because they are so prone to injury. They can't play alone or with other children because they are so easily injured. Like autism, the cause and best care for their illness is unknown, so Khadija must work with a condition that medical professionals do not fully understand. Khadija told me that her doctor has told her: "We can't help." Khadija's children face a lot of social alienation, so she needs to support them through their emotional struggles.

Molly asked Khadija if she wanted to hear what Molly had written, and Khadija declined. Khadija's application cycled through two more rounds of review and resubmission because the administrators asked for further medical documentation. Molly contacted Khadija each time, and Khadija arrived at Midnimo with the plastic bag. Finally, Khadija's application was rejected because the condition could not be approved as a "related condition." Molly called Khadija to relay the county's emailed rejection.

After the rejection, I went to Khadija's house with Warsame, a newer case manager at Midnimo. Khadija welcomed us with weary regard. Khadija's husband and three children were home; her 13-year-old son Muse, for whom Khadija was seeking services, was sitting on the couch watching TV, and the other children were in a different room. Warsame's and my aim was to take photos of all potentially pertinent documents. This way, we wouldn't have to keep asking Khadija to return to Midnimo with the plastic bag. As we took photos, Khadija spoke, with Warsame's intermittent translations, of her children's medical journeys. She had first sought care for them in Arizona, and they now saw doctors at two different hospitals. She said they went to the hospital multiple times a month, but nothing helped. She wanted to see a specialist, but the wait lists were never-ending. Warsame asked Khadija how things were going at school. At the change in topic, Muse, who had been ignoring us in favor of the TV, demanded to know why Warsame was asking about school.

"That's not what you're here for," Muse told Warsame in English.

We stopped talking about school and took photos in silence. When Muse left the room, Khadija told us that Muse was bullied every day at school. In Somali, she said, "He's retaliating now, telling the bullies he'll kill them. Now he must be searched by administrators every day. He hates school. He refuses to go; he's missing so much school." Before she could say more, Muse returned to the room, and Khadija said only, "Thank you for any help."

I didn't know it at the time, but that afternoon of repetitive photo-taking and cut-off conversations would mark my last meeting with Khadija. Khadija did not return to Midnimo, and she did not return any of Malyun's, Molly's, Warsame's, or my text messages or calls. On one end, this departure was just that, a departure, silent and unknowable, a lost story. Absent not only from the county's records but from this study is Khadija's voice. Khadija brought in a plastic bag of institutional documents to speak for her. Khadija delegated all WCAG writing to Molly. Khadija removed her voice from the grant process. In place of Khadija's voice, I have medical documentation and field notes, Molly's earnest but failed attempt to repackage Khadija's story into a fundable proposal, and six numbers, the end date of Khadija's participation.

But, as rhetorician Cheryl Glenn (2004) has argued, silence is not passivity; silence is not rhetorical emptiness. Silence can also be "a space of possibility, an untapped reservoir of energy, that beckons attention as a rhetorical art" (Smilges, 2022, p. 84). The position that rhetoric happens through writing and speaking, through public communicative acts undertaken by agentive rhetors, obscures much rhetorical action from the margins, where publicity isn't always safe (Johnson and Kennedy, 2020) and where testimonial injustice muddles the voices of many (Fricker, 2007). In some cases, then, "absence becomes a rhetorical strategy, a way of making meaning when conditions would otherwise render it impossible" (Smilges, 2022, p. 25). Khadija's absented voice and her departure are not necessarily voids but are also instantiations of "rhetorical absence," a signifying silence, "a lacuna that harkens to meaning found elsewhere" (Smilges, 2022, p. 5).

Elsewhere, there are Khadija's unopened medical records, her arrival without any medical documentation, her ambivalence about securing a new diagnosis for her children, her disinterest in the language Molly used to describe her children's health histories. These stances are not exclusively signs of lacking medical knowledge. They are also positionings of oneself as apart from institutions and their knowledge. They are turnings to care and meaning elsewhere. Elsewhere, too, there is Khadija's initially optimistic participation in the WCAG program, her talks with other mothers, her trips to Midnimo with her medical document bag in tow, the time she brought her children to spend time with other children whose mothers were in the program. These were labors invested in the work of weaving medical resources into community care. Many participants, like Khadija, recalled first seeking disability services because their children were "different" or had a "sickness," often "our community's sickness." As Khadija told Molly, she arrived at Midnimo that October morning because her friend had told her "to come to Midnimo because they would help parents with sick kids" (1/22/2018). Somali mothers like Khadija gathered based on shared experiences of community sickness—of supporting their children as they endured bullying, violence, and racialized surveillance at school, of supporting other each within costly healthcare systems, of navigating the intricacies and dead ends of state services. When Malyun sent WhatsApp messages about the WCAG, mothers who identified as having a sick child and needing help flocked to Midnimo, a grassroots organization known less for their specialized expertise than their creativity in pooling resources to help Somali women. The meeting room was abuzz with hope. Elsewhere, there was community sickness, biosocial care coalitions informed by the shared experience of community sickness, and informal networks of mothers helping mothers survive systems that were never designed with their lives in mind.

By contrast, the WCAG's reliance on medical diagnosis recategorized children by diagnosis and divided coalitions of mothers along diagnostic lines. The WCAG application necessitated that its parent-authors co-write a new, medical story of a child's body, health, care, and future. In response, Khadija's absent documentation and departure refuse to reform collective, all-Somali networks of care and understandings of autism as community sickness. Eight fellow mothers' rhetorical refusals also opted out of diagnoses that would break up groups formed on a basis of shared experiences of community sickness and redistrict a community of care into diagnosis-based, private patient-provider dyads.

Refusal 2: Disclosure (4 Participants)

The second site of rhetorical refusal, disclosure, occurred when applicants were asked to answer questions about family life and health and to then invite county assessors into their homes to verify their written answers. In response, some mothers expressed wariness about how the personal information they wrote into their applications might circulate and ultimately hurt their children. At this juncture, four mothers enacted rhetorical refusal as a protective enclosure against state surveillance, even if that surveillance came with resources. Sofia's story, which takes place at the intersections of confidentiality, racialized surveillance, deficit-based models of disability, and autism stigma, depicts this rhetorical refusal. When Sofia, a Somali American mother of two who worked as a registered nurse at a large hospital, sat down with Nimo, a community health worker, to write her WCAG, Sofia led with her concerns about confidentiality: "I have a four-year-old son, Isse, and he has autism. And the one thing I should say before we start is that confidentiality is really important to me. My husband is not OK with the diagnosis. For now, we don't talk about it. Family members don't know about it. We don't talk about it with anyone" (2/15/2018).

Nimo assured Sofia that their meeting was confidential, and Sofia agreed to continue with her WCAG. Sofia had arrived with full medical documentation, and the application process moved quickly. Sofia wrote on her own until she reached the question "Are there significant behavior disturbances affecting family life?"

Here, Sofia exclaimed, "My son has only been diagnosed for eleven months, and already I've answered this question so many times."

Nimo prompted Sofia with examples of how she could answer the question ("Does he get upset if you change a routine? Does he run away?"); Sofia clarified that it was not that she did not know how to answer but that she did not like the way that the application assessed her son: "Sometimes I want to think about his strengths." Sofia then offered a story to speak to those strengths and to the stories that applications like the WCAG gave her no space to tell. Sofia narrated: "You see, my older daughter has trouble relating to Isse, so I try to really talk about my son's strengths—or, not even, just, like, how he's enjoyable as a person. Like, when my older one does a scanty job washing her hands, I'll say, 'Oh, you're doing an Isse wash, huh?' And she's like, 'What?' And I say, '*you know*,' and I mimic how Isse washes his hands, just very not well, and then my older daughter laughs and laughs, and Isse laughs and laughs. And they pretend to wash their hands together. And she says, 'I'm doing an Isse!' And I just point out things, like, 'Doesn't it make you smile when Isse does that?'"

In the WCAG, the applicant's narrative was instrumental to getting approved for funds. The WCAG asked how a child might "disrupt family life." The WCAG evaluated a child's disability in relation to other household stressors, described as "single parent, family size, loss of job, other family members with disabilities, low income." Disability, like unemployment and divorce, was grouped as one more blow that a family might endure. Social service staff encouraged parents to emphasize the stressful elements of their children's autism because the more stress they could enumerate, the more resources they could qualify for. Anisa, who was a parent of two children with autism and had successfully enrolled in long-term services and now helped other parents do the same, described the process of enrolling in services as one of telling negative story after negative story about your own child: "What you have to do is, every month, you tell the state what's wrong with your child. You list everything that's wrong with them, all the ways they're a burden and all their struggles, and then you do it every single year again and again" (5/27/2018). Some parents, like Sofia, were not willing to craft stories about their children's negative, stress-inducing qualities. Parents generally wanted resources, yes, but that did not mean parents were willing to craft stories about their children in purely transactional ways. The stories parents told about their children mattered. They mattered in ways other than how these stories could recoup funds. Applicants like Sofia cared about the stories they told about their children, the ways they described their children, even to faceless audiences. And they were not willing to reduce a child to a list of burdens.

Further, the qualities that the WCAG marked as burdensome or stressful were not universally experienced in these ways. The behaviors marked as burdensome and therefore worthy of disability compensation tracked a phenomenon that anthropologist Julie Livingston (2005) describes as "why and how the lack of certain capacities or bodily configurations can trump the possession of others in social life" (p. 8). The WCAG marked dependency as not normal, as disabling, stressful, and improvable. But few Somali American mothers saw dependence as a necessarily bad state in need of correction. Before returning to Sofia's story, consider this discussion between Kowsar, a Somali American mother and WCAG applicant, and Molly, a Midnimo community health worker who was assisting Kowsar with writing her initial WCAG. The two discussed the same WCAG question that asked a parent to list the behavior disturbances affecting family life, in the following conversation:

KOWSAR: No. There are no disturbances.

MOLLY: Well, but, what things are hard because of autism? Like, are there foods he won't eat? Or times he runs away?

KOWSAR: I see my son as a blessing. He teaches me. Through him, I've learned about autism. I learn through him. He teaches me how to be a parent.

MOLLY: Can you remember a time that there was conflict, though? Even if it was ultimately good. Like, you learned from it?

KOWSAR: He has gotten so much better because of my younger son. My younger son comes home from daycare, and he just wants to talk to his brother, and my youngest son says to me, why doesn't he talk? I say, it's ok, he has speech delay, you can talk to him. He sits here [balls fists under chin and slumps], and my youngest son just, la la la, and my oldest son, I think this helps him, and he has gotten better.

MOLLY: That's so great. And so, they have fought before?

KOWSAR: No.

MOLLY: OK, but it sounds like speech delay, with your older son, right? Not speaking?

KOWSAR: Yes.

MOLLY: So, speech delay for sure. And that makes it hard to communicate in the family? One sibling having to take on a lot more responsibility, maybe?

KOWSAR: [nodding]. (2/3/2018)

This was how Kowsar's unfundable story of siblings finding each other on their own terms was rewritten into a fundable story about a stony older sibling and a younger sibling tasked with too much. Kowsar was led to narrate her older son's lack of speech and his interior nature as problems, burdens, rather than as parts of his personality that his family enjoyed and respected. Kowsar was coaxed to package her son into a deficit-based story exchangeable for state support.

As Kowsar's and Sofia's stories depict, Midnimo and social service staff often had to coax Somali mothers into telling stories about their children that were grounded in deficiency. But participants' reticence to provide the state with a deficit-based story about a child was compounded by and inextricable from their precarious positions as racialized immigrant mothers whose admissions of struggle might get translated not into funds but into punishable accounts of unfit parenting. County workers often instructed parents, when answering questions on a disability application, to describe a child "on his worst day." This strategy, a social service professional told me in an interview, helped ensure that the parent would get approved for the maximum number of resources for which she was eligible (2/1/2018). Participating Somali American parents, however, reported fears that describing a truly stressful day may make the parent appear incompetent and could compel the evaluating social worker to report a mother to child protective services (CPS). Participants explained that they, as Black, immigrant mothers, some of whom were not fluent in English, some of whom were in the process of applying for citizenship, were not granted the same good faith that white mothers enjoyed. Bodies of research, journalism, and activism have documented the racist, punitive impact of the child welfare system and its power to investigate and separate families (Roberts, 2001, 2022). Somali American applicants did not relate to the state as a neutral, privacy-honoring entity, as was assumed by the WCAG application and its probing questions. One participant confided that her former PCA had reported her to CPS, and seven participants told stories of mothers they knew who had been reported. One participant explained, "The first time he [my son] ran away, I was by myself. I didn't know what to do. I called 911. I thought they would take him from me. You hear people talk about it all the time" (2/2/2018). Another participant explained: "My biggest stress in the day is being at the bus stop on time. If I'm not at the bus stop, what would they do? Hopefully the bus driver wouldn't let [my kids] off, and would take them back to school, but if that happened: Would they could get taken from me? Would I be arrested?" (3/25/2018). These stories suggest that the felt threat of state surveillance and criminalization was real, one that shadowed everyday acts of parenting and one that loomed over the WCAG's requests for disclosure.

In Sofia's meeting, Nimo, as she had been trained, urged Sofia to shape a story of her life with her son as stressful. After Sofia told her story about Isse and the joyful handwashing, Nimo responded, "It's just to get help with funding. It's just to get music and swim lessons, you know?"

Sofia nodded and waved her hand into the air, as if to say, *I know it's silly*. She reached for the pen and wrote: "He gets upset when we have to go out of a normal routine. Hates loud noises. Doesn't play with others" (2/15/2018).

Before Sofia left the meeting, though, she asked Nimo if Nimo knew what would happen if Sofia's son was evaluated by the State Medical Review Team (SMRT), a prerequisite for any long-term aid. Sofia asked if her son's teachers would see his SMRT diagnosis. She wondered if the diagnosis could be reevaluated. Sofia explained that she did not want her son's autism diagnosis to be the first thing his teachers learned about him.

"Sometimes I do worry," she confided, "that my husband's right. On one hand, I know he's not, and Isse needs help, but I also think, maybe Isse will start talking when he's ready. Look," she showed us a picture of her son's smiling face popping out of a balloon pit. "My husband always says, he's late-blooming, like his uncle." In this aside, Sofia sought to genealogize autism, like the health literacy students did in chapter 1. Sofia recontextualized her son's negative diagnosis as a valued family trait, and one that would change and grow as her son changed and grew. She did not want this negative label to block out the positive elements of her son's autism and character.

Nimo told Sofia that she believed that SMRT evaluations could be reevaluated at regular intervals. However, she wanted to make sure that she gave Sofia the right information. "Let's hold onto your application," she told Sofia. "Then I'll talk to the people at Human Services. Then I'll call you, OK?" The following week, Nimo went to social services with Sofia's questions. I was at the meeting when Nimo asked Sofia's question to Amanda, the social service professional who also worked as a WCAG evaluator. When Nimo reported Sofia's worry that "a SMRT diagnosis would stay with her son forever," Amanda cut Nimo off with the firm statement "Well, I am of the belief that no one grows out of autism." Nimo persisted and eventually got Amanda to explain that SMRT evaluations are redone every five years, but Amanda seemed short and dismissive for the rest of the meeting.

Amanda seemed to perceive Sofia's question to be indicative of a scientifically erroneous belief, one that holds that autism can be cured. Amanda's dismissal of Sofia's concern as unscientific illuminates the difficulties of communicating concerns about health in bureaucratic processes and to institutions, wherein scientific-medical discourses are the sole expert discourses (Lay, 2000). This encounter depicts another instance of testimonial injustice (Fricker, 2007) and rhetorical disability (Owens, 2013). Amanda instantly heard Sofia's concern as one caught up in antiscience beliefs that autism is a Western disease that can be cured. In other words, when a Somali parent pointed out the problems built into the WCAG—for example, when Sofia expressed concerns about a diagnosis compounding discrimination for a Black boy at school, or when a parent pointed to potential legal impacts that loomed for Somali American mothers if they were to put into writing the stresses of parenthood—she was dismissed as scientifically illiterate. These silencings depict, once more, how medical illiteracy is wielded to delegitimize "unneeded or unwanted knowledge" (Dorpenyo, 2022, p. 305), particularly when that knowledge is spoken by a racialized person and undercuts a "stock story" that "people in dominant positions collectively form and tell about themselves" to keep power relations neutralized and in place (Martinez, 2014, p. 36). Amanda's hasty response—"I am of the belief that no one grows out of autism" (2/20/2018)—rewrote Sofia's deeply informed and protective uncertainty as a wrong belief. Sofia's disinclination to put her son's diagnoses on state and school records was not a sign that she misunderstood autism, was not a sign that she thought her son might be cured, and was not a sign that she was ashamed of her son or his diagnosis. Sofia's concern was informed by "experiential and embodied knowledge of people of color [that] is legitimate and critical to understanding racism that is often well disguised in the rhetoric of normalized structural values and practices" (Martinez, 2014, p. 35). Sofia's wariness about the WCAG application and the SMRT evaluations, and the ways these documents would ink an autism diagnosis onto her son's lifelong record, was informed by her lived experience of racist and ableist norms that she had encountered in her son's schooling and elsewhere. Sofia imagined that a formal diagnosis would bury her son's strengths and his unique personhood and would make it easier for teachers to underestimate him. But in the social services office, Sofia's concerns about privacy, surveillance, and stigma at school were swiftly rewritten as errors, indicative of lacking health literacy at best or as antiscience, backward beliefs, at worse.

Nimo, however, was not deterred by Amanda's dismissal and obtained the information her client needed. Even with this new information, Sofia did not submit her WCAG. Sofia explained in a later interview that she kept her application in her purse for weeks and continued to attend Midnimo's workshops, but because Isse was working with a speech therapist at school and doing well, Sofia decided to follow her husband's lead and wait. Like her family members, Sofia worried that a deficit-based diagnosis would not fairly represent her son. In the county's records, Sofia's nonaction, the application at the bottom of her purse, was coded as an absence. One of the twenty applicants that failed to secure funds.

But as a rhetorical refusal, Sofia's unsubmitted application resists the WCAG's grounding definitions of disability and the application's imperviousness to the reality of racialized surveillance and autism stigma. The questions required Sofia to describe her son in terms of burden. Writing a child's story to the state as one of burden was trying enough, but these requests for stories of stress brought real, racialized danger to Somali families in the US. Autism diagnoses threatened to expose children to more discrimination at school. Stories of parenthood's stress threatened to expose mothers to state surveillance and punishment. Hemmed in by these discourses and structural threats, parents could not tell the stories of their children in the pages of the WCAG. "To be visible," Johnson and Kennedy (2020) have written, "especially as a person from a marginalized community, is to 'summon surveillance and the law'" (p. 162). Here, public rhetorical strategies like speaking and writing are unsafe, and rhetors adapt other means of communicating. Absences, silences, and mistakes emerge as viable rhetorical strategies, modes "of making meaning when conditions would otherwise render it impossible" (Smilges, 2022, p. 25). Rhetorical refusal helps recognize these silences not as fixable mistakes but as participatory, meaningful, protective, and resistive actions.

As a rhetorical refusal, Sofia's unsubmitted document signifies loudly. It illuminates and rejects the assumptions that disability is a burden and that funds must go to whomever can write the story that frames a child as the most burdensome. It calls attention to the uneven risks that deficit-based storytelling and state verification of such stories bring for mothers of color. Equipped with a lived knowledge of the state's power to weaponize children and threaten families, refusals like Sofia's are rhetorical. They are informed by exigences of racialized surveillance and legacies of family separation. They are informed by the reality that in applying for social services, Somali American mothers must put themselves in a structurally vulnerable positions. Rhetorical refusal, as a concept, surfaces this counterstory, voices Sofia's lived knowledge as legitimate, and vibrates with meaning behind the blank space next to Sofia's case number in the county records.

Refusal 3: The Fundable Plan (5 Participants)

The prior rhetorical refusal showed that the WCAG application requested that applicants report on a child's dependencies as family stresses, a line of questioning that implied that the more assistance a child needed, the more eligible a family was for funding. Yet, as participants submitted their applications, it became clear that WCAG funding was not awarded based exclusively on need but also on applicants' abilities to write a fundable plan. The grant administrators denied all but two of participants' initial plans. According to evaluators' criteria and instructions, approvable plans requested medical therapies or disability-specific aids that could measurably help a child become more independent. When grant evaluators rejected applicants' plans, applicants were invited to resubmit their applications. However, upon receiving rejections, five applicants left the program rather than resubmit a plan. These departures, as rhetorical refusals, reject medicalized care for children as well as the underlying assumption that caregiving should push children toward a standard type of independence. As rhetorical refusals, these unfundable plans and departures gesture toward care that would help a child thrive, rather than fit every child into a mold of measurable self-sufficiency.

The final page of the WCAG asked applicants to request services or goods, to describe how these services or goods "are related to disability," and to demonstrate that their requested services or goods advanced a care plan that was "sustainable." After each question, there were three inches of white space. Grant administrators told applicants that it was fine if they handwrote their responses. No preparation, drafting, or polish necessary. Lynn, a Wingham County staffperson, explained in a meeting with a Somali applicant, "In this section, you want to write your plan, what you want. This section isn't going to be your case manager's plan, or your county's plan, or your doctor's plan—it's going to be your plan" (2/22/2018). However, the ways in which WCAG evaluators assessed applicants' plans demonstrate that there were, in fact, unstated rules. In my analyses of parents' applications, county responses, and WCAG evaluators' criteria, I identified four unstated rules that parents had to follow to be approved: (1) parents had to request services related to a medical definition of disability, and services had to be grounded in medical evidence (i.e., no experimental treatments or alternative medicine); (2) parents had to request services that fell into the jurisdiction of social services to fund; (3) services could not fall under what social service professionals called the "typical parent responsibility"; and (4) plans had to be designed to measure a child's improvement toward independence. I discuss these unstated rules in the remainder of this section and then address why some applicants responded with rhetorical refusal.

First, requested services had to respond to medically demarcated, disability-specific needs. The following explanation, offered by a grant administrator to a Somali American parent who was confused about why her request for tutoring had been denied, represents the social service approach to determining whether a plan is disability-specific enough:

> These grants work in two parts. They're supposed to be bridge grants, so just a little bit of money while you're waiting for longer services to get approved. [. . .] The grant has to provide something enriching to your child, and that something has to be related to disability. So, something that is hard for your child to do *because of* his disability. For example, maybe he can't take a swim lesson because there are too many kids and noises, but he could take a private swim lesson or a swim class for kids with autism. That second part is important: it can't just be any swim lesson. It must be for kids with autism. Look for things like "sensory-friendly." (3/23/2018)

To be successful, applicants had to request services or goods that were necessary because of a child's medically defined disability. When it came to assessing WCAG proposals, grant administrators repeatedly explained that all fundable services had to be institutionally sanctioned forms of caregiving: medically validated, cost-effective, and disability-specific.

By contrast, Midnimo-recruited parents imagined diffuse and family-wide benefits from their possible WCAG funds; parents requested funding for nonmedical, not disability-specific services. Maryan said that she was going to take her three children on their first vacation. They planned to go to Boston, the city her son loved but had never visited. Kadra planned to take her daughter to Kenya and visit her ailing mother. Nasra wanted to help her son do better in school and was eager to learn about private tutoring. Nasra's friend, coaxed to come along to the meeting, related that she hoped to send her child to a summer enrichment program. Ilhan requested money to help pay rent, as her family had experienced many unplanned moves in the last year. Four mothers envisioned a return visit to Somalia, where they hoped healers could provide their children with religious treatments and reinvigorate the children's relationship to Islam. The most common applicant requests were educational assistance, such as after-school tutoring (10 applicants), help with rent and groceries (8 applicants), a trip to see family (8 applicants), and assistance with behavioral, speech, or occupational therapy (5 participants). None of these requests were approved. There were usually several reasons that these requests were denied, but a key reason was that Somali applicants often asked for resources (rent, food, family recreation or travel) that would help their entire families as a unit, while the WCAG could only fund services that related to a discrete, medically endorsed, autism-related need.

A second and related reason for denials of the above requested services was that many of these services did not fall into the jurisdiction of social services. Four applicants, for example, had their requests for tutoring denied. When Annelise came to one of Midnimo's WCAG workshops, one parent asked Annelise why her request for tutoring had been denied. Annelise admitted that, yes, she could see how it might seem like tutoring should be funded, but that when "you work in the county, you come to learn that everything gets divvied up into specific categories. Tutoring is the responsibility of the school system or, of course, the parent, but not social services" (3/1/2018). In interviews, Somali parents identified one of the most frustrating features of the American healthcare system as its specialization—participants were frustrated that they had to seek out so many different and uncoordinated medical professionals to care for different aspects of a child's health. Siloed specialization also characterized social services, the successful navigation of which required an understanding of what institutions cover what kinds of needs. Showing how disenfranchising these specialization-dependent systems can be, Decoteau (2021) has argued that "because historic systems of care have not been fully reconfigured in the contemporary era, those who 'misfit' into autism's landscapes of care (on the basis of race, class, and impairment) fall through the cracks between the categories of mental health and developmental disability, and between the institutions of education and medicine" (p. 70). For Somali American participants, being "trapped between [. . .] institutional silos" meant participants' plans were rejected because they requested services outside of the grant's silo.

Ayan's story helps illustrate how these often-unstated rules could derail parents' requests, even when these requests were in line with the spirit of the WCAG. Ayan was a single mother of three children with multiple disabilities, and, at her first WCAG consultation, Ayan told her community health worker, "I need a bed and a stroller."

"Okay," said Muna, who was working with Ayan. She wrote down these items. "Can you explain why?"

Ayan had her explanation ready: "For the bed, I need an enclosure or a whole bed with an enclosure. One of the beds that would keep him inside. Because I wake up in the middle of the night because Mohamed gets out, and he's downstairs getting into things, breaking things. He could hurt himself. I bring him back up, and it happens again. I don't sleep. The other two sleep through the night. And the stroller. Right now, I can't bring them anywhere because they would run out into the street, or they would run away. Like Ede? I can never go because how would I bring my kids? They wouldn't stay put; they would run away. People say, Come! Bring them! I say, I know my boy. If he doesn't want something, he will get on the ground, yell, attack. I have never gone to Ede. I can never go to any kind of social thing because what would I do with my kids?" (3/15/2018).

On the surface, Ayan's requests aligned with the WCAG's mission. They were single items that would help Ayan's children with a disability-related need while also allowing Ayan a bit of respite—she would get a full night's sleep and enjoy community events with her family. But Ayan's plan was denied because neither item was disability-specific; Ayan had requested a large stroller and a zip-up tent for a bed, neither of which was designed specifically for people with disabilities. As well, Ayan didn't have the proper documentation to support that her children needed strollers for mobility. Finally, the county assessors were concerned that these items didn't move Ayan's children toward greater independence. Ayan's plan was denied, and she left the WCAG program.

Third, social service staff referred to the rule called parent responsibility factor to demarcate services that were beyond any sort of state fundings. At the Midnimo meeting where Annelise explained that tutoring was outside of the purview of social services, Annelise went on to outline how this question was a good opportunity to talk about some of the ways that applicants could write successful plans; she explained that it comes back to the parent responsibility factor. I use this to explain what services we will and will not cover. The parent responsibility factor is basically an assessment of what is a typical parent responsibility and what is above and beyond a typical parent responsibility. So, if you're asking for money for a typical parent responsibility, like feeding your children, then social services will not do that. If you're asking for money for something that is above and beyond, that is disability-related, that is adaptive, then we can cover that. So, we can't pay for you to go on your family's road-trip vacation, but we can pay for you to get adaptive equipment to take your child on a vacation.

The parent responsibility factor positioned the application as a tool to evaluate how well parents were fulfilling their responsibilities—and not to support parents' lived knowledge of what their families needed. Thus, when participants requested help with rent or a trip to Somalia because participants had deduced that these measures would support their families, grant administrators overruled these requests as both the parent's own responsibility and as outside the silo of social services.

Lastly, even if plans were medically endorsed, related to disability, and beyond the state-approved typical parent responsibility, these plans had to be grounded in metrics. To write a successful plan, applicants were taught to write quantifiable goal-setting plans that would document how requested funds would measurably alleviate a disability-caused burden. Lynn explained to parents at Midnimo how to set goals for a child and relate these goals to fundable activities:

> So, you identify what you need: a behavior therapist, a music therapist. Then, list the goals you are going to make happen. How will this staffing help this person with autism become independent in the community? You start with a long-term goal. Then you break that long-term goal, that big goal, into little steps. Then, you make the little steps measurable. Your plan needs measurability. How are you going to make sure that this person you're paying is doing the job that they're supposed to do? What this all means for you is that you need to write a chart, and then, when you're filling out the charts, you really want to focus on explaining why the staff you're hiring meets a need of your child's and how this need is related to your child's disability. (3/23/2018)

Lynn then reassured her listeners that "when you think of this whole process, you should really think that it's easy. It's easy because you know this person best, you know this person and what they want. You know what you want to ask for. Really, you know everything that you need to know, so now you're ready to go home, fill this out, and turn it in tomorrow" (3/23/2018).

Later in the WCAG process, a different WCAG administrator showed me an example of an accepted WCAG proposal and its description of activities. It read:

- Goal: Joy will have appropriate social skills (Long Term Goal).
- Objective: Joy will increase social skills by engaging in a weekly play activity with a peer. (Short Term Goal).
- Action Plan: Staff will take Joy to the community center once a week to play with peers. Staff will model and teach turn taking with Joy prior to the community outing. Staff will model necessary steps to the activity and encourage her to try. Staff will praise Joy for each attempt at trying to interact with her peer and displaying appropriate behavior.
- Measure: Joy will interact with a peer for at least 5 minutes while playing.
- I need these services because: Joy can play next to a peer but not interact. Joy needs staff to model appropriate behavior and social cues.

This prioritization of goal-setting illuminated how the WCAG process shored up disability as a medical deficit, but one that could be improved with a plan. At the time that I read this example, I was holding the following proposal, which was written by a Midnimo-recruited applicant. In its entirety, it read: "The funds will be used to hire after school tutoring to prepare him for graduation. The services will help one child get the help he needs to graduate." The WCAG funding process was designed to facilitate activities that promoted self-sufficiency, accountability, and measurable goal-setting. Lynn's well-meaning assurances that Somali parents already knew everything they needed to know depended on her incorrect assumption that these values were universal. By contrast, Somali American applicants often requested funding that would support collective networks of care. Somali American applicants often sought funding to support their family's functioning as a unit, often a globally dispersed unit (rent money, family vacation, trip to East Africa). These requests failed.

Somali American applicants' unfundable plans and departures disengage from the state's definitions of disability, parenting, and caregiving. The WCAG's trail of unfunded proposals shows that the rhetorical situation into which parents wrote their WCAG applications was undergirded with unstated cultural norms, including a medical understanding of disability, a prioritization of self-sufficiency, and an alignment with medical expertise. Underlying the WCAG's person-centered premise was the assumption that all applicants would ascribe to logic of "compulsory able-bodiedness" (McRuer, 2010) and its related "pathologized dependency" (Teston, 2024). For these reasons, the WCAG put many Somali American mothers into a double bind. The rhetorical work that mothers had to undertake to gain material resources that the WCAG promised (behavioral therapies, money for caregiving, even an autism diagnosis itself) came at the expense of cultural, community, and social resources. To write a successful WCAG application and to then use funding in approved ways, parents had to disentangle themselves from caregiving networks based on shared experiences of community sickness. Parents had to seek out clinical diagnoses and individualized behavioral therapies for their children. Parents had to surveil, measure, and report back on their children's progress. Parents had to mold their children toward norms of independent adults. Some parents refused these terms.

Within the WCAG application-writing and evaluation processes, parents' mistakes—incorrectly written plans, missing goals and metrics, absent documentation, requests for unfundable services—are not necessarily mistakes but can signify as rhetorical refusals. These mistakes, silences, and departures were a means of rhetorical participation in a structured, top-down space of communication. One way that applicants articulated dissent was through their unfundable plans. In writing their unfundable proposals, Somali American applicants not only rejected the state's terms of disability and care and the underlying logic of "pathologized dependency" (Teston, 2024); applicants also made their needs plain. Mothers described for their state interlocutors exactly what good care and real support looked like for their families. They voiced the importance of one-on-one educational tutoring, of having stable housing, of food security, and of keeping children connected to their culture, religion, and family around the globe. Somali mothers showed up and told the county what care would look like for them. Even though the WCAG allowed only for "institutionally productive means of talking" (Keränen, 2007, p. 179), Somali American applicants' mistakes, these poignant visions of care, remain on the record. These mistakes, as rhetorical refusals, insist on possibilities that the WCAG rendered unsayable, unfundable, illegible. These mistakes, as rhetorical refusals, leave traces of what a different kind of public aid could provide. These wrong answers, as rhetorical refusals, arc toward supports that directly respond to the conditions of community sickness—tutoring to help at school, rent money to help with housing instability and chronic evictions, funds to visit home. These wrong answers were not funded, but as rhetorical refusals they illuminate problems that need redress. They also illuminate concrete solutions that would help families. Mothers' unfunded and unrevised plans stand as rhetorical refusals to assimilate to the county's standards of good parenting and as unyielding commitments to their knowledge of what their children need.

Refusal 4: Tracking Care (3 Participants)

If awarded, the WCAG required grantees to keep and submit records of how they were using funds. At this juncture, three parents secured funds for respite caregiving but were then dropped from the WCAG because they did not follow reporting procedures. Four out of six funded applicants settled for the WCAG's most easily acquired service: a one-time $600 payment for informal caregiving. Applicants could secure the $600 check if they committed to using the money to pay a caregiver to stay with their children while the parent engaged in respite care. The WCAG asked that participants who were awarded funding for informal caregiving nominate caregivers who were appropriate and credible in the eyes of the state, justify pay for their caregivers based on industry standards, and record the caregivers' working hours and completion of assigned duties. Participants who received the $600 check had to submit documentation with the name, contact information, and relationship of the caregiver, along with a signed statement that this person had not been convicted of a crime and was over 18 years old, and had to document each time they paid someone to provide caregiving. Parents also had to write a list of goals that the caregiver and child would work on together and justify how these goals advanced independence and socialization.

These requirements were necessary for the county's own reporting requirements, but they also asked that parents invite more surveillance into their homes and, further, that parents act as surveyors themselves. Reporting requirements asked parents to rewrite trusting, reciprocal, and long-standing relationships into transactional and tightly bounded ones. At this juncture, one mother did not submit the required information for the county to perform a background check on her appointed informal caregiver, her sister. The other two applicants repeatedly turned in incomplete time sheets for their appointed caregivers, who were also family members. In this final section, I argue that these three participants rejected the WCAG's reconfiguration of trusted care networks into state-mediated transactions. Participants enacted rhetorical refusals against caregiving grounded in surveillance and transaction as well as broader economic devaluation of care work.

The WCAG's documentation requirements, even for the $600 caregiving fund, proved disruptive to participants' lives and inconsistent with their values, such that three participants gave up the funds that they had devoted so much time and labor to secure. Ilhan, who was rejected for incomplete time sheets, joked with a community health worker and me that the reporting required by the WCAG canceled out its promise of respite: "They want me to record her [my niece's] hours, what she did to help [my son], am I babysitting the babysitter?" (5/1/2018). The reporting rules often disrupted families' existing relationships, care practices, and daily rhythms—all while inviting more domestic surveillance into family's homes. Anthropologist Annemarie Mol (2008), writing about the shift in healthcare to promote individual choice and patient self-direction, has argued that "introducing patient choice into healthcare does not (finally) make space for us, its patients. Instead, it alters daily practices in ways that do not necessarily fit well with the intricacies of our diseases" (p. 2). The WCAG's reporting procedures were part of the WCAG's consumer-driven structure, but these procedures "alter[ed] daily practices in ways" that situated parents to adjudicate over transactional caregiving relationships. To further illustrate this final refusal, I offer three short examples that show how the WCAG reorganized caregiving relationships into employer-employee exchanges.

The first example illustrates how the WCAG allowed for specific and contingent ways of using support staff. At a Midnimo WCAG workshop, Annelise described different professionals whom Somali parents, as potential grant recipients, should use to coordinate their state funding:

> If, or when, you get a grant, and if you go on to get a waiver, you're going to get a new case manager no matter what. You will have an annual assessment done. Your case manager will work with you in a crisis, will consult with you if you need it, will monitor your current plan, authorize services, and assist you. Then, you need to select a fiscal support entity, or an FSE—we refer to them as banks or accounts payable—but you have to pick one, and they'll provide monthly spending reports, and they make sure everyone gets paid. They handle all taxes and payroll. Rule number one: never contact your case manager about payment. Always call your FSE. Never call your FSE in a crisis. Call your case manager. We like clear boundaries. (2/9/2018)

Annelise identified specific, functional entities that parents should employ. Annelise described each role, case manager and fiscal support entity, as bounded and specialized. Grantees should not call their case managers with financial questions, just as they should not call their fiscal service entities in a crisis. These were not relationships that a parent could build, develop, and learn to trust. These professionals functioned as siloed tools. As tools, these professionals were also contingent. Annelise opened her remarks by clarifying that when applicants switched social services, they would also switch case managers. These relationships were temporary, tied to specific tasks, and interchangeable. Everyone—parent, case manager, fiscal support entity—functioned independently, self-sufficiently, and according to a circumscribed role.

The second example shows how person-centered grants required that applicants rewrite family relationships along transactional lines. Consumer-directed grants, including the WCAG, were unique in that they allowed parents to employ themselves, family members, or other selected persons as PCAs. This affordance was a huge draw; in many cases, family members were already working as full-time caregivers, and now they could be paid for their quintessential caregiving. Parents could keep care work in the hands of already trusted people. However, what was less apparent were the rules that family caregivers would have to follow. Lynn explained to parents how they should manage their selected support staff:

> Some important points: minimum wage is $12; maximum wage is up to $18; and parent or spouse pay is up to $17.40 an hour, and that does include payroll taxes. You all know the legalese in this: "up to." Remember, this is a budget. You need it to last. You need it to meet all the needs of the person you're here for. A brother or sister may say, well, I can get paid up to $17.40, so give me $17.40. What PCA gets paid $17.40? *None*. You want to start at that lower amount, $13.00 an hour. At the end of the year, there's a raise, so account for that. Pay really must be based on knowledge and skill. You're not going to pay the same amount to someone who got fired from Burger King the same as someone who has worked at a nursing home for two years. (2/22/2018)

Lynn warned participants not to pay kin more than they would a professional. Lynn instructed participants to remap familial support to match budgets, industry wage standards, and employment incentives. Market standards come from a system in which women earn less than men, and women of color earn less than white women. In this model system, care work is severely devalued such that those working in the care sector struggle to make livable wages. Nonetheless, Lynn clarified that this was the model to follow. And further, the skills a family member might bring as a caregiver—such as a long-term relationship with a child and parent, familiarity with the household structure, trust—were not monetarily valuable. Pay must be tied to standardized credentials.

The third example demonstrates how the grant required ongoing surveillance—here, parents themselves acted as go-betweens who surveilled their appointed caregivers, who were often trusted family members, and reported back to the state. Jenn explained why it was important to record the hours that a paid support person worked:

You want to make clear that you have a plan to make sure the person you hired is actually doing the job they're hired to do. So, this chart is here for you. It helps you. Think about this: say you have people over for a football party, and everyone is grabbing food and drinks from the fridge, and you have your staff there to watch your child, and your staff starts work at 9 p.m. Then, it's 9:05 p.m., and your staff is grabbing food out of the fridge for a snack. This chart can help you. You can say, hey, look at this form we both signed, we agreed that you start work at 9 p.m. If you want to change the contract and start at 9:30 p.m., OK, we can talk about that, but right now, your contract starts at 9 p.m., and I'm not paying for you to grab a snack. So, this chart really is for your protection. (2/22/2018)

Jenn spun the reporting as a boon for parents: "It helps you," Jenn insisted, meaning that careful recording would help the parent by ensuring accountability. Jenn's examples painted care providers as untrustworthy. Unsupervised, they would slack on the job. Unchecked, they would badger parents for more money. In the social services model, everyone functioned as an individual looking after their own best interests. Consequently, parent-employers needed to be vigilant and tightfisted. Even if parents did not see their paid caregivers in these punitive ways, the grant's reporting procedures positioned parents as meticulous managers and their paid care staff as under surveillance. Relationships that might have depended on reciprocity, trust, distributed agency, and collective responsibility for caregiving had to be rewritten to fit within a privatized economy of monitored relationships.

In response to these rules, one grant recipient did not follow the background check requirements, and two recipients submitted incomplete time sheets; when asked to correct these mistakes, all three recipients left the program—with money on the table. In the institutional communication arrangements, there was little recourse to raise concerns with or ask for alternatives to these reporting procedures. In unilateral, bureaucratic communication structures, you're either following the rules or you're making mistakes. In turn, mothers' mistakes—unsubmitted documentation and incomplete time sheets—make arguments within these top-down, one-way communication structures. Mothers' mistakes disrupt the circulation of power through communication, through rhetoric (Dolmage, 2014, p. 2). At this fourth juncture, three mothers refused to rewrite their relationships along individualized, transactional lines. Their refusals rejected transactional, documented relationships as the bedrock of care. As rhetorical refusals, these parents' departures leave in their wake meaning, leave in their wake an unspoken but nonetheless articulate insistence upon the possibilities of other, less regulated, and not inherently suspicious models of care and compensation.

Rhetorical Refusal in Institutional Documentation

The WCAG program fell short of its aim to enroll Somali American applicants in their microgrant and to bridge families into long-term services. Ultimately, 20 out of the 26 Somali American applicants left the WCAG program with no services. One way to respond to this result is to fold the program's failures into the frames of health literacy and cultural competence. In these frames, Somali American applicants were not literate enough—in medicine, in science, in bureaucracy—to correctly complete the forms, and county administrators were not culturally competent enough to localize their services to Somali American applicants. In these frames, solutions are premade: more literacy education for Somali Americans and more cultural education for social service professionals. There is truth to these explanations and value to their proposed solutions. But they are only part of the story.

Following applicants' mistakes, silences, and departures as rhetorical refusals tells a crucial counterstory about what went wrong and what could be different. Somali mothers' rhetorical refusals in the WCAG program, enacted through mistakes, silences, and departures, demonstrate how important, as well as how easily dismissed, rhetorical refusals can be in top-down, institutional processes. In the WCAG, the applicant told her story by answering the form's questions and providing the requested evidence. Applicants provided personal information about employment, marriage, divorce, health, and daily family stressors. In return, applicants received form letters from the county notifying them if their application had been accepted, denied, or had led to requests for more information. To verify the information that applicants provided, case managers would come to their homes and observe their families. If the applicant was successful, there was more surveillance and reporting in store. Throughout, there was little space for dialogue, and any dialogue required that the applicant navigate automated help options and wait in long lines. Writing about the delivery of healthcare, rhetorician Rachel Bloom-Pojar (2018) has explained that "if the goal of a program is to provide healthcare to a community, then the language used to discuss health and illness must reflect the discourse of that community" (p. 57). Such was not the case for the WCAG—and is rarely the case in bureaucratic processes. Because communication is top-down and regulated and because institutional languages and community languages about health rarely intersect, rhetorical refusal is a crucial way for applicants to participate, argue, and make discursive space for other possibilities within institutional writing and communication situations.

To demonstrate the intransigence of institutional documents and communication structures—and to thereby highlight why rhetorical refusals are a vital communication mode within institutional documentation—I turn to rhetorician Lisa Keränen's (2007) study of one hospital's "do not resuscitate" (DNR) worksheet, as this study conveys just how airtight institutional documents can be. Keränen studied a DNR worksheet developed to support patient autonomy in death. The document asked the patient to manage their death by selecting what interventions they wanted and did not want. The DNR worksheet seemed to invite the patient to make choices and prescribe plans for medical professionals to follow, but Keränen peels away this veneer of agency and shows that by naming and thereby delimiting the patient's choices, the document assumed hospital and technological death and precluded consideration of alternatives. The patient could choose which interventions (defibrillation, ventilation, tube feeding) they wanted, but the patient could not question the premise of the document, which was that death was a hospitalized, technologically mediated event. The DNR worksheet allowed patients "to (think they can) choose (how) to die" (p. 200).

Uncapping a pen before the WCAG, a Somali American parent-applicant was in a similar position as the patient checking boxes on the DNR worksheet. In the WCAG, applicants could voice the specific stresses their families endured due to autism, but they could not articulate autism outside of a deficit-based framework. Applicants could choose medical services, but they could not suggest nonmedical care. Applicants could identify their own goals for a child, but they could not do away with goals altogether. Neither could applicants question whether independence was a goal that made sense for every child. Applicants could select and pay a caregiver, but they could not allow that caregiver to work without supervision and outside of industry pay standards. The WCAG assumed dominant valuations of disability, self-sufficiency, expertise, and parenting and *then* asked: What resources do you need to pursue these ends? If the applicant wanted to discuss any of the WCAG's premises and built-in choices, there was little recourse to do so—just long waits on hold and form letters. In response, some parents enacted rhetorical refusal.

Rhetorical refusal is one tactic that form writers can use to resist the underlying logics that structure institutional documentation, such as the DNR worksheet and the WCAG proposal. In these uneven, hierarchical communication spaces, rhetorical refusals—blank answers, wrong answers, incomplete applications—are one of limited rhetorical means to participate, speak back, and communicate outside of the document's allowable stories and demanded confessions. Rhetorical refusal is useful to both make visible and disrupt the "institutional voice" (Keränen, 2012) and the unstated sets of assumptions that undergird institutional documents. Rhetorical refusals are "strategies marginalized subjects deploy to be recognized on their own terms" (Yam, 2019, p. 3), even if those terms render them ineligible for public aid. Blank forms, unreturned documents, and departures are rhetorical activities that "generate meaning from absence and the ways people on the margins of society tap into these potentialities in order to build community, navigate hostile spaces, and resist forms of institutional and state-sponsored violence" (Smilges, 2022, p. 4). In such nondialogic, tightly regulated discursive spaces, rhetorical refusal is one of the few agentive moves possible for a rhetor to talk back to institutions.

As rhetorical refusals, what do applicants' mistakes, silences, and departures communicate? Applicants' rhetorical refusals unsettled the underlying, deficit-based logics of the WCAG, logics built on specific and ableist protocols about parenting. Parents' rhetorical refusals concretize some of the imaginative work that Eli Clare (2017) has described as crucial to living in a world of interdependence, rather than one where we all must strive for measurable independence; Clare writes, "In conjuring a world where we need care to get up in the morning and go to bed at night, we picture an overwhelming dependency, a terrifying loss of privacy and dignity. We don't pause to notice that our fears reflect not the truth but the limits of our imagination" (p. 136). Mothers' unfundable plans, metric-less futurities, and blank answers do not lack for imagination but, instead, describe what on-the-ground interdependence looks like in their families and could look like with additional resources and support. Rhetorical refusals leave behind fragments that articulate other ways of conceiving disability and interdependent practices of parenting and care. At the first site of refusal, mothers refused the ways that diagnoses fractured their biosocial collectives into private, clinical relationships. Mothers showed up at Midnimo because they identified as needing help, but they did not see a diagnosis as the right trail to follow to that help. There were other ways, the absent diagnoses averred, to respond to their children's needs. Second, mothers left silences or wrong answers when the application probed at the stress their children brought to family life. These blank answers, unsubmitted applications, undisclosed stressful days, and missed caseworker appointments formed a protective enclosure around their families, an enclosure that insulated them against surveillance, against deficit-based assumptions about disability, and against standardized aims for children.

At the third juncture of refusal, mothers did not propose plans that sought to fix or improve a child's disability. Their wrong plans—missing goals, proposing clearly unfundable services—described care aimed at supporting a family as a unit rather than intervening to correct specific deficits in an individual child. Instead, these unfundable plans asked, what if we cared for a child's present-day thriving over their progress toward a singular, neoliberal model of successful adulthood? What would that kind of care and government support look like? Mol (2008), in advancing her deeply contextualized "logic of care," has developed the term "patientism" to refer to the experiences of patients, healthcare providers, and others working together to "explor[e] ways of shaping a good life" (p. 47), to "craft more bearable ways of living *with*, or *in*, reality" (p. 53). There is no singular or linear or diagnosis-standard way to chart such a course; rather, in Mol's logic of care, patients and providers "do things," they try out different practices, consider what works and what doesn't, and continually adjust (pp. 90–94). This logic of care is "first and foremost practice. It is concerned with actively improving life" (p. 103). Somali American mothers, in writing their care plans, posited practical ideas that could improve their lives, that could help them provide good care in the actual, lived contexts of their day-to-day lives. Applicants described how rent assistance, individualized support at school, after-school activities, or a vacation would help their individual children with autism *and* would help their families. Their plans did not respond to a specific diagnosis and its standard, medical care practices; rather, their plans considered a diagnosis in its sociohistorical, material, political, embodied, and cultural contexts, and they sketched models of care that responded to these contexts.

Fourth, mothers refused to rewrite caregiving as a transactional, low-paid service, wherein providers and clients were at perpetual odds. These rhetorical refusals, communicated through incomplete time sheets and missing documentation, envisioned care that operated on trust rather than surveillance. Across all four refusals, mothers refused to tell the stories that the applications requested, stories wherein their deficient children brought stress that could be improved with professional, metric-driven, evidence-based interventions. Mothers' mistakes, silences, and departures made space to care for children in ways that were not legible within the terms of the WCAG.

While county evaluators, bound to their criteria, rejected these proposals, there nonetheless remains a record of how state funds *could* support these now-departed families. This record is documented in blank spaces, incomplete answers, delinquent time sheets, missing documentation, and handwritten care plans. Reading these rejected proposals through the lens of rhetorical refusal connects the dots between these silences and brings into focus refusal's arc and its rhetoricity. Mothers wrote about how they could use help with rent and groceries, tutoring at school, travel funds to help families stay close across diaspora, and vacations to bring families rest and joy. These so-called mistakes depict that participating parents had little interest in disability-specific resources that were geared at making a child more independent. Mothers sought resources that would connect a child to communities they valued—school, family, and religion, for example. Mothers sought resources, such as consistent housing and food, that would make family life more secure.

Mothers abandoned the program when they were met with requirements for surveillance—assessor visits, charts to document a child's progress, and time sheets to use to track caregivers. Participants' mistakes and rejected proposals envision investments in existing communities. They envision supports not predicated on moving a child measurably from dependence to independence. They envision care plans that do not have to be justified in writing, grounded in evidence of stress, endorsed by professionals, tracked through measurable goals, and reported in terms of caregiver hours and tasks. Written off as remediable mistakes, these stories disappear. Heeded as rhetorical, participatory, and meaningful refusals, they cohere and communicate; they signify and argue; they arc toward a different terrain of public aid.

Conclusion

The WCAG was described as a small grant. The program was a stepping stone to long-term services. The application was short; the evaluation process, streamlined. Ideally, the WCAG would be forgotten as soon as its original class gained more substantial support. When the WCAG's partnership with Midnimo did not meet its stated goals, again the WCAG was described as a minor misstep. It hadn't worked for these families, but it had illuminated barriers, such as low health literacy and language barriers, that could be addressed in a future iteration. This chapter has told a different story of the WCAG, one that should not be explained away. The grant empowered norming discourses about care, disability, health, and parenting. The grant abstracted questions about these topics from their contexts—for example, there was no consideration of how reporting a stressful day at home could bring different consequences depending on a mother's skin color, hijab, or language background. In response, Somali mothers refused to play by the WCAG's rules that they submit to new layers of surveillance and regard their children as projects to mold toward independence. Applicants' mistakes and silences—an unfundable service; a blank space where an applicant should list the family's stresses; a time sheet with only rough estimations of clock-in and clock-out times—are rhetorical refusals to buy into state-sanctioned practices of disability and care. Parents refused definitions of disability grounded in deficit. Parents refused notions of care that were built on surveillance and specialization. Parents refused the drive to make a child normal rather than support them. These refusals were rhetorically generative. Many parents, as this chapter has shown, paused in dictating their application to talk about their children in ways that the WCAG interface did not allow. These rejected applications therefore envision a new kind of public aid. The next chapter follows five mothers who departed the WCAG and entered a new domain of care, one grounded in theories of the human microbiome and one that supported some of these visions of care, disability, and health that parents' WCAG refusals arced toward—even as microbiome healthcare led parents further and further away from the stability and benefits of evidence-based medicine.

CHAPTER 4

The Persuasive Microbiome

Rhetorical Refusal through Care

Rhetorical refusal unfolds along an arc. Rhetorical refusal's "no" grows from fertile ground and acts in service of yet-unrealized futures. As Benjamin (2016) wrote, refusals in medicine can be "seeded with a vision of what can and should be, and not only a critique of what is" (p. 970). What futures does "no" make possible? What happens after someone refuses what, they are told, is the only right decision? What's next? This chapter engages one future that opens in the wake of rhetorical refusal. In this chapter, the "what's next?" is the microbiome. Five mothers who left the WCAG program found support under the care of naturopaths who defined autism as an illness resulting from an unbalanced microbiome and who prescribed care through diet, outdoor play, relocation, and other alternative, often experimental treatments. For participating Somali American mothers, these microbiome models of health and illness offered causal explanations of autism that aligned with their beliefs about community sickness and opened for them agentive, collaborative subjectivities in relationship to their children's healthcare. Whereas the previous three chapters have followed Somali parents' rhetorical refusals in relation to the broadly generalized futures they envisioned, this chapter examines a site of refusal at which mothers were building concrete futures through material practices that responded to the overlapping exigences of community sickness. The resulting care was not perfect, and in this chapter, I also consider how microbiome etiologies of autism exposed parents to predatory experimental treatments and cut parents off from medicine's benefits, even as these benefits are unevenly distributed.

This chapter begins with an examination of twenty-first-century scientific and popular texts about the human microbiome. I show how authoritative microbiome discourses advance a deeply contextualized human body, one whose health cannot be considered on its own but only in constant relationship to other bodies, environments, and experiences. And yet, even as microbiome literature describes a biosocial body enmeshed in its environments, much microbiome care focuses on individualized, probiotic interventions in ways that obscure these very environments, including social determinants of health and disease. For these reasons, microbiome innovations respond to and advance the needs of the privileged. But this mainstream narrative is not comprehensive, and people from positions of marginalization do indeed use, adapt, and innovate microbiome discourses and practices. The second part of this chapter explores the experience of five Somali American mothers who remade scientific and popular microbiome discourses in their relationships, care routines, concepts of identity and belonging, and etiologies of autism. Participants' everyday acts of microbiome-informed caregiving materialized a future where experiential knowledge is valued, care is collaborative, and disability caregiving is not oriented toward the braided goals of self-sufficiency, normalcy, and progress. The microbiome lent a scientific (or pseudoscientific) vocabulary to the distinct ways participants described autism as community sickness. Across participants' accounts of the microbiome, I identify five topoi, or commonplace categories, that engendered participants' distrust of medicine and allegiance to the microbiome. These topoi illuminate why microbiome care meshed with participants' daily lives and belief systems. Beyond this study, these topoi offer a portable framework to recognize and respond to medical dissent as rhetorical refusal. These topoi serve as tools to identify discrete sites at which health knowledge sentiments in people's lives. It is at these sites where knowledge can mesh or repel, that trust can build or break down. This framework is useful to both better understand why people turn away from medicine—one of the guiding questions of this book—and to identify starting points for medicine and public health to better fit with people's everyday lives, constraints, values, and concerns.

Who Is the Microbiome For? Popular and Scientific Discourses of the Microbiome

A shopper sees a strawberry yogurt with the label "probiotic and low-fat," thinks, "That sounds healthy," and drops a few yogurts in his cart.

A pediatrician suggests to a pair of concerned parents that they try incorporating probiotics like yogurt and fermented foods into their child's diet as a first line of defense against the child's undiagnosed stomach pains. "Live bacteria = gut health," one parent jots into their notebook.

A lab tech feeds a rat inulin-included drinking water. Next, the rat will be mated and have offspring. The offspring will be surgically investigated to learn whether consumption of inulin during pregnancy alters maternal intestinal microbiome composition. This finding could help scientists understand if a mother's microbiome makes her offspring more likely to contract asthma.

A baby's pacifier falls into the dirt at the playground; the mother picks up the pacifier, hands it back to her child, and says, "This'll help you get a strong immune system, Bug. No daycare colds for you!"

The above are moments of microbiome discourses at work. They gesture to the breadth of microbiome discourses; microbiome discourses get taken up by microbiologists conducting federally funded studies, parents trying to piece together different sources of health information, and marketing teams charged with selling more wellness products. The human microbiome is buzzy, exciting, and mysterious; it is an increasingly popular topic in both scientific research and popular culture. Federal funding initiatives, magazine articles, best-selling books, TED talks, diet trends, and health and wellness products have all arisen around the microbiome. Science journalist Ed Yong, in his 2016 book *I Contain Multitudes: The Microbes within Us and a Grander View of Life*, positioned the microbiome as the "most significant revolution in biology since Darwin" (p. 15).

The "human microbiome" refers to the trillions of microbes that make up a human body. The microbiome is in a constant state of flux, always evolving in relation to its environments. For these reasons, the human microbiome could transform our understandings of the body, the self, and our relationship to our social world. And yet, even as the concept of the microbiome seems well positioned to advance more socially embedded understandings of health, disease, and human interconnectedness, studies and related media coverage of the human microbiome often atomize structural causes of health and health disparities. This section summarizes scientific and popular discourses of the microbiome published between 2008 and 2018, a ten-year span during which research about the human microbiome was expanding and gaining attention. I show how microbiome studies and media coverage define and discuss the human body and its health and then focus on how these texts often aspire to a postracial future of personalized medicine, while, in their application, much microbiome care focuses on individual interventions in ways that obscure the social determinants of health and disease. Microbiome applications tend to frame complex, multifaceted health problems—for example, malnutrition, chronic illnesses, mental illnesses—as caused by individual microbe imbalances and as treatable with probiotic interventions. As with most seemingly new medical discoveries, the microbiome gets folded back into status-quo ways of thinking about the body, particularly in terms of disability, race, and gender.

"Only 10% Human": Microbiome Definitions and Metaphors

The human microbiome refers to all the microorganisms—bacteria, fungi, viruses, archaea—living within a human body. In each person, the microbiome consists of 10–100 trillion microbial cells, each with its own genetic material (Ursell et al., 2012; Marchesi and Ravel, 2015; Gilbert et al., 2018). The human microbiome is essential to life functions. Microbes produce vitamins that human genes cannot produce on their own. They break down food and extract nutrients. Microbes teach human immune systems to recognize pathogenic microbes and develop anti-inflammatory compounds to fight them off (NIH Human Microbiome Project, 2012). Microbiome research endeavors to understand the role that these diverse symbiotic microbial cells play in the human body and their impacts on human health. The NIH's Human Microbe Project set out to map human microbiota; the project has produced 5,177 microbial taxonomic profiles, but the aim of mapping a common healthy microbiome has proven unlikely, as microbiota are so responsive to their environments that it might be impossible to document a standard healthy microbiome (Yong, 2016).

Illustrative of the microbiome's profundity, much popular and scientific coverage of the human microbiome starts with the premise that the human microbiome is large. Abundant, teeming, populous, complex, vast. Longtime *New York Times* health columnist Jane Brody (2017) described the microbiome as composed of "trillions of bacteria, viruses, and fungi that inhabit virtually every body part, including those tissues once thought to be sterile." A review of human microbiome research led with the following definition: "We coexist with vast populations of microbial species that make a host out of the human body. It has been estimated that up to 100 trillion microbial cells make a home out of us, and likely outnumber human body cells by an order of magnitude" (Mulle, Sharp, and Cubells, 2013, p. 337). Relatedly, the ecosystem is a dominant metaphor for the microbiome. The human microbiome is widely framed as a fluctuating, permeable ecosystem populated by millions of microbes pursuing their individual and colonial self-interests, all in symbiosis with other microbes. Once the invaders of human health and bodily integrity, bacteria were now maintainers of its ecosystem. This idea that the body is a porous ecosystem populated by microbes destabilizes the concept of a singular self sealed within a body. Science writer Michael Pollan (2013) claimed that the day he learned of the microbiome was the "exact" day that he switched to "think[ing] of [him]self in the first-person plural—as a superorganism, that is, rather than a plain old individual human being." Geographer Jamie Lorimer (2017) has described this new kind of human as an "unraveling halobiont—a multispecies chimera that is kept alive, sane, and rational by its microbes," and has reiterated that this kind of human "unsettles the modern idea of health as the absence of microbes and of the human as a mind in a vat" (p. 4). "We are," as Pollan (2013) wrote, "only 10% human."

"An Impoverished Westernized Microbiome": Illness in the Microbiome

A microbiome understanding of the body's vulnerability to illness represents a departure from traditional germ theory and its depictions of the human body as a closed entity to be protected against germs (Martin, 1994). Microbiologists Michael Toh and Emma Allen-Vercoe (2015) cautioned readers that the microbiome might come as "somewhat of a shock to those of us who were raised to think of all microbes as 'germs' to be eradicated" (p. 265). Center the microbiome, and dysbiosis, not an invading germ, becomes the foundational concept of disease. In early life, birth (cesarean or vaginal), infant feeding, diet, and exposures to antibiotics seed an infant's microbiome. From there, diet, antibiotic exposures, and adaptation to one's environments shape the microbiome (Toh and Allen-Vercoe, 2015). Microbiome research often associates sanitized, indoor environments with depleted, unbalanced microbiomes. Thus, Western, domestic "hygiene regimes" (Rook, 2012)—washing hands, cleaning surfaces, using antibacterial cleaning supplies—that have been normalized as practices of good health are recast as unhealthy, misguided labors that have created too-clean spaces and have depleted their inhabitants' microbiota. In 1989, David Strachan's hygiene hypothesis posited that the runaway success of Pasteurian approaches to germ warfare made many of us too clean. By the early 2000s, Strachan's hypothesis had been developed by other immunologists and microbiologists into a biome-depletion or disappearing-microbiome hypothesis, one that explained that exposure to "old friend" bacteria was an important but disappearing part of healthy microbiome constitution (Rook, 2012); human microbiomes in many Western, postindustrial countries were depleted, and, as a result, populations were encountering a suite of chronic, noncommunicable diseases (Blaser, 2014). These "epidemics of absence" (Velasquez-Manoff, 2012) include autoimmune, allergic, and inflammatory diseases such as asthma, type 2 diabetes, eczema, food allergies, and neurological disorders including autism. Regarding autism, some microbiologists have posited that autism may not be a "static, inheritable neurodevelopmental disorder" but a "dynamic system of metabolic and immune anomalies involving many organ systems, including the brain, and environmental exposure" (MacFabe, 2015, p. 52; Kang et al., 2017). In line with the idea that environments and experiences can balance and set off-balance the highly responsive microbiome, there is another, specific risk to the microbiome: human migration. Immigration to the US is associated with a loss of microbiome diversity and is compounded over generations (Vangay et al., 2018). Western migration depletes the microbiome and increases risk, especially over generations, of developing chronic diseases, even relative to individuals born in and continuing to reside in their Western countries of origin (Vangay et al., 2018).

In sum, microbiome research and journalistic coverage have centered birth, infant feeding, and early diet, especially antibiotic use and exposure, as pivotal events for establishing a baseline healthy or unhealthy microbiome. From there, key experiences such as immigration or antibiotic exposure, as well as a culmination of mundane experiences such as diet, office work, or "dirty thumbs or dog licks" (Pollan, 2013), shape the microbiome and, in turn, shape human health. The next subsection accounts for on-the-ground practices that individuals take up to balance their microbiomes, many of which rely on essentialized notions of global North and global South lifestyles.

"Rewilding": Managing the Body as a Microbiome

Based on the premise that the human microbiome is depleted by everyday activities typical of living in Western, postindustrial places, many microbiome-focused interventions aim to diversify the microbiome by reengaging with premodern practices. As Pollan (2013) wrote, "researchers now speak of an impoverished 'Westernized microbiome' and ask whether the time has come to embark on a project of 'restoration ecology'—not in the rain forest or on the prairie but right here at home, in the human gut." Many microbiome therapies happen at the DIY level, with microbiome enthusiasts testing out their own treatments, from conservative, like making homemade kombucha, to extreme, such as consuming hookworms or orchestrating fecal transplants. Efforts to replenish the microbiome are often called "rewilding" efforts, to indicate that healthy microbiomes harken to a premodern time when hygienic environments and overprocessed foods weren't a thing.

Popular texts and marketing campaigns have advanced this vision of a rewilded gut and have outlined steps to make one attainable. Prominent microbiologists have released popular science books that pathologize the Western microbiome and promote probiotic, natural lifestyles, under titles like *Dirt Is Good* (Gilbert, Knight, and Blakeslee, 2017) and *Let Them Eat Dirt* (Finlay and Arrieta, 2016). Popular health magazines broadcast probiotic diets, and marketing campaigns highlight probiotic properties of foods, like the number of active cultures in a yogurt. Microbial medical interventions include personalized medicine, probiotics, prebiotics, and diets designed to match and enhance a person's microbial and genetic makeup, such as human-derived microbial strains or next-generation probiotics (Gehrig et al., 2019). As with many health-related initiatives, microbiome therapeutics target and are most accessible to members of the upper class, those with money and time to pursue extracurricular health projects. For example, a few high-end childcare facilities have advertised the lengths they go to ensure children encounter dirt and reap its benefits; there are daycare centers that have installed forest floors composed of dirt, berries, mosses, and shrubs to fortify children's microbiomes (Molteni, 2020).

Other microbiome-inspired health interventions happen in underground spaces, where individuals united around health problems test microbiome interventions on themselves. Lorimer (2019) has studied individuals who reseed their microbiomes by introducing hookworms into their bodies. Lorimer's scholarship focuses on people who have chronic autoimmune conditions, who have faced disappointments in medical care, and who have found helminthic therapy online. Lorimer describes a microbial therapy that has served as a lifeline for people with marginalized, poorly understood, or underresourced conditions. These individuals have formed their own networks of care based on iterative self-experimentation and pooled knowledge. Together, though, these diverse practices, from paying extra for dirt to keeping tabs on probiotic strains to delving into the underground world of hookworms, attest to the diverse "therapeutic possibilities of managing the human as a microbiome" (Lorimer, 2019, p. 67).

"Ghost Variables": Gender and Race in the Microbiome

Gender and race are rarely discussed outright in microbiome literature; the vision is that microbiome care is so personalized that gender and race are nonfactors (Newkirk, 2016). But this idea of medicine so individualized that gender and race can be transcended is usually a fiction. Because microbiome discourses rarely consider the interplay of gender, race, class, ethnicity, and health, microbiome-informed care risks neutralizing and perpetuating health disparities.

Above, I explained how the initial composition of the microbiome happens intergenerationally, through vertical transmission, but also individually, at key, early life moments, including birth (cesarean or vaginal?), infant feeding (breast or bottle?), and early diet (how processed?). These sites and associated practices are gendered ones that center the mother; as such, microbiome discourses risk evolving into another scientific discourse used to medicalize and moralize women's lifestyles and decisions. As scholarship about the medicalization of pregnancy, childbirth, infant feeding, and mothering has shown, when maternal activities are deemed medically beneficial, then these activities become medically endorsed, urged, documented, surveilled, and, at the same time, removed from the maternal body and from a mother's social, lived contexts (Koerber, 2013). As vaginal birth, breastfeeding, and avoidance of antibiotics are situated as practices that promote an infant's microbiome health, so, too, do mothers become responsible for these health practices and culpable for not optimizing them. In the US, even if mothers are equipped with this knowledge, many encounter structural barriers to having vaginal births, breastfeeding their children, proffering a wholesome diet, and avoiding antibiotics. American mothers live in a country where one out of three women will have a Cesarean birth (the rate is highest for Black women), where many new mothers have limited healthcare resources and limited to no paid parental leave to support them to breastfeed, and where many parents cannot afford to stay home with a sick child and therefore need antibiotics to keep their children in childcare and school. American children receive, on average, between ten and 20 courses of antibiotics before they turn 18 (Blaser, 2011). Increasing amounts of antibiotics also lace meat, milk, and surface water (Kumar, Arnipalli, and Ziouzenkova, 2020). Even as microbial research describes a body inextricable from its environment, applications of microbiome science abstract a mother from her social context. These social contexts often stymie a mother's attempts to have a vaginal birth, breastfeed her baby, prepare healthy meals, and avoid antibiotics. Putting microbiome science to use is impossible for most American mothers.

To similar effects, racialization and systemic racism also remain largely absent from microbiome research and clinical applications, such that anthropologist Amber Benezra (2021) has termed race "a ghost variable" across human microbiome research because this research often bills itself as a postracial precision medicine, a claim that all but guarantees unexamined categories of race will surface in pernicious ways. To clarify, race is a social category, not a biological category, but race categories are important to the study of medicine because the lived experience of race and racism affects how racial difference is scientifically made, studied, and verified; how health disparities form; and how care is delivered (Roberts, 2011). The microbiome is no exception.

Race in microbiome research is further complicated by the fact that much of the research itself benefits from systemic racism and its role in sustaining scientific research. Much microbiome research leverages colonizing histories and racialization processes. Following a history of exploitative medical research practices, some microbiome research has approached Indigenous populations in the global South as "ready bodies for microbiomic explorations" (Benezra, 2020, p. 882). Such microbiome research "bioprospects" (Hayden, 2003) the microbiota of Indigenous peoples and takes the knowledge to profit researchers, corporate backers, and well-heeled Western populations for whom "a healthier, non-western microbiome could become a matter of buying bacterial cultures" (Stallins et al., 2018, p. 161). Related criticism has shown how microbiome research practices can rely on and thereby reify racial categories and assumptions. While microbiome science aspires to a postracial precision medicine, research participants are often grouped by race and ethnicity; there are "Westerners' who are primarily white and are assumed to have similar lifestyles versus black and brown bodies in the global south assumed to be underdeveloped or 'modernizing'" (Benezra, 2020, p. 882). These sociohistorical categories get neutralized as evidence to demonstrate biological differences between "industrialized" and "traditional" microbiomes. Such explanations of difference assume biological differences between these constructed population groups but do not account for the colonizing scientific histories as well as current economic, political, and social contexts that shape health differences. Rhetorician Kelly Happe (2013) has argued that biomedical discourses in genetics and epigenetics can ontologize race through a rhetorical strategy of disavowal and recuperation; scientific literature will disavow race as not a biological category—as in, claiming race is a social construct outside of the purview of good science—but then recuperate race as an explanatory factor for persisting health disparities. Health outcomes are then attributed racial identity rather than social conditions. Such frameworks endorse biomedical solutions that respond to problems in individual bodies rather than social solutions that aim to reform systems.

Demonstrating how race is disavowed and recuperated in microbiome research, Benezra (2020) has analyzed a much-cited, NIH-funded microbiology study that connected preterm birth in African American women with specific vaginal microbes (Fettweis et al., 2019); this study was followed by a study to reduce African American women's preterm birth risk with targeted interventions to biologically modify their microbiomes (Ravel and Brotman, 2016). Undermining this neat probiotic solution is much research showing that the chronic stress endemic of living within racist structures contributes to higher rates of preterm births among African American women (Villarosa, 2023). Instead of addressing structural causes of health disparities, "millions of dollars are being used to fund studies of microbes in the vagina, trying to fix the problem of preterm birth by fixing a broken vaginal microbiome" (Benezra, 2020, p. 887). It is, again, the "magic bullet model of disease" (Scott, 2003, p. 221), the technical solution that "function[s] structurally and rhetorically as ways of avoiding addressing the systemic problems that cause [disease]" (Lawrence, in Welhausen et al., 2015, p. 9). In this case, microbiome interventions molecularize race on the level of the microbe (Duster, 2006) and thereby atomize structural causes of race-aligned health disparities.

In sum, the progress of microbiome research has depended on colonial, racist, and exploitative geopolitical relations; the benefits of microbiome research have clotted around the white and wealthy Western world; and microbiome applications further bracket these same structures by disavowing race as a category relevant to science and then recuperating race at the microbe level to atomize race-based health inequities. Anthropologist Heidi Paxson (2012) has argued that microbiome-informed care does not harken back to a premedical past or open to a post-Pasteurian future but rather uses a familiar combination of scientific evidence and neoliberal assumptions about personal responsibility to broaden the purview of medicine and the individual responsibilities of the good health citizen. Health practices that might seem to be opposites—for example, carrying hand sanitizer everywhere versus paying a premium for a dirt-floored daycare—are locked into similar codes of neoliberalism, individualism, and health citizenship. The focus remains on individual health optimization and not on structural changes needed to address health disparities.

Who Is the Microbiome For?

So far, this chapter has examined popular and scientific discourses that describe the microbiome. Here, the microbial body is one that dissolves boundaries, as the environment, the social world, and day-to-day activities change the trillions of bacteria that make up the human microbiome and that change us from the inside out. While this contextualized model of human health has radical potential, microbiome discourses often operate in normalizing ways. They moralize health along gendered, raced, and classed lines, and they advocate technical (probiotic) solutions to complex social problems. Too, and as with most health innovations, microbiome practices are most available to the elite, those with the money, time, and means to learn about and procure microbiome health tools. At the same time, just because white, affluent people are constituted as the desired users and default agents of microbiome science and care does not mean that they are the only ones creating, using, and adapting microbiome discourses and practices. Much in the same way that antivaccination beliefs get cordoned off to wealthy and white parents, such that parents of color and parents of lower socioeconomic classes are seen not as antivaccine agents but as ill-informed and underresourced parents who just need access to better information (my argument in chapter 2), so, too, do the discourses of the microbiome elide the potential agency of anyone who is not white, Western, and wealthy. In popular microbiome discourses, much like discussions of vaccine hesitancy, the white and affluent are positioned as agents of microbiome knowledge-production and care. Marginalized people are positioned as either outsiders to microbiome practice or as the passive victims, the people to whom microbiome research happens or the people who do not have the requisite privileges (money, literacies, connections) to avail themselves of its benefits. But racialized and marginalized persons are not just acted on by microbiome science. Microbiome discourses and therapeutics get taken up by those who are marginalized—just not in ways that are widely legible.

Few studies have asked how marginalized persons relate to, understand, and use the microbiome, its discourses, and its therapeutics, experimental, alternative, or medical. Nonetheless, microbiome epistemologies, discourses, and tools are taken up in inventive and protective ways by not only affluent, white wellness aficionados but also by many less-heard others, including Somali American mothers in diaspora. For some Somalis in Minnesota, etiologies of the microbiome were useful in that they supported their beliefs that autism was a Western disease (Decoteau, 2021), one that occurred in unique ways for Somali children because of their displacement and social marginalization. The microbiome lent scientific validity to many mothers' conceptions of autism as community sickness. The human microbiome, like community sickness, did not deal in abstracted disease entities and sealed-off bodies. Somali American parents' arguments that migration, health disparities, food production, diet changes, hospital childbirth (longer hospital stays, cesarean births, use of antibiotics), and abrupt exposures to new pollutants, technologies, lifestyles, and medicines made their children susceptible to autism are all given scientific credibility within microbiome theories of autism. The next sections follow the stories that five Somali American mothers told about the microbiome and autism. These stories speak to the protective, healthful, and adaptive ways participating mothers used microbiome discourses and practices.

Nasra's Story

The following two sections engage stories about how five Somali American mothers adapted microbiome understandings of the body and autism to guide their family care practices. These sections are informed by the words of the following five mothers:

- Asha, four children, including two boys (12 years old and 14 years old) diagnosed with autism
- Asma, four children, including a nine-year-old girl diagnosed with autism
- Farah, three children, including a seven-year-old boy diagnosed with autism
- Layla, three children, including a five-year-old boy diagnosed with autism
- Nasra, three children, including a six-year-old boy diagnosed with autism

This section opens with Nasra's story, excerpted but told in her own words. Nasra's story depicts an experience common across all five mothers' stories; Nasra narrates how medical modes of knowing autism chafed against her family's routines, values, and shared futurities, while microbial modes of knowing autism meshed with family life. I begin with Nasra's story because her account speaks to the granular, lived experiences of medical and microbial modes of knowing autism, and I then analyze related patterns across participants' stories.

Nasra arrived in the US as an 11-year-old girl. She was born in Somalia but had spent most of her childhood in a refugee camp in Kenya. She arrived in Florida with her mother, moved to South Dakota, and then to Minneapolis, where Nasra's mother had fewer personal connections but had heard that the schools and services were much better than those in the Dakotas. Nasra enrolled in community college, where she planned to study to become a registered nurse. She was elected as president of the college's Somali Student Association and, from that time on, found herself positioned as a leader in her Somali community. When I met Nasra, she had recently earned her master of arts degree and worked at a university, where she taught cross-cultural health communication classes to, as she described it, "so many white boys in baseball hats. They grew up on farms. They look at me like, whaaat? But we find our common ground" (4/15/2019). Nasra also worked with Midnimo as both a consultant and client. Midnimo hired Nasra as a consultant to plan and lead workshops, and Nasra participated in Midnimo autism-related workshops. For our first formal interview, I met Nasra at her office; Nasra's primary job, in addition to her teaching and consulting, was as a program director at a Somali-run nonprofit focused on helping Somali parents navigate the public school system. Nasra had three children, an eleven-year-old daughter, Zakia, who was present for our first interview, during which she perched on the edge of Nasra's desk and completed schoolwork; a six-year-old boy, Zeki, who was recently (ten months ago) diagnosed with autism; and an 18-month-old boy, Hassan, whom, Nasra told me, she feared would have autism, too. "It's our community's sickness," she said, "It happens to our boys, and his brother," she shrugged, as if to indicate the diagnosis might be a foregone conclusion.

At the beginning of our interview, Nasra directed my attention to a matte photo of Nasra and her three children pinned to the carpeted wall of her cubicle. She told me, "When I thought about this talk, I wanted to start with this picture. It was the end of another hard week, and we got dressed up, went to the mall, and we posed, and we took these photos. The baby was almost a toddler. Everything was rushing on, and I wanted to have these photos. We were all happy, everyone behaved.

"The next day," Nasra told me, "Zeki got his diagnosis."

It seemed clear that Nasra had planned for our interview. She had charted how she would tell her story, what pieces she would bring forth, how she would organize and attach meaning to events. My role was to listen. In the remainder of this section, I include Nasra's story in three excerpts. The first part describes Zeki's developmental assessment, the second part describes a state case manager's visit to Nasra's home, and the third part describes a typical appointment with Nasra's new naturopath. The first two sections are excerpted directly from our interviews, and so consist of Nasra's own words; the third is told as a combination of field notes and interview transcripts.

1. The Assessment

"Zeki's assessment wasn't supposed to be the next day. We had two months until his scheduled assessment. It wasn't supposed to be until January 20th. This day will forever be in my memory. January 20th. Every day I checked the appointment time because I can't miss it. Every morning I log into the website, check the time, make sure it's still the time I think it is. I have it in my calendar, I have it in my packet of papers, and I have it on my phone, but I am so anxious that I'm going to forget it. Sometimes I think, Do I have the same thing Zeki has? Do we share this condition?

"But they had a cancelation, so they called down the list, and I was the one who answered and could make it. When I got the appointment, I booked us a motel room. I thought we should be close to the place, like physically close. I found a cheap place, forty dollars. The appointment was in the morning, and I didn't want anything to go wrong. If anything went wrong, we would go all the way to the end of the list, we wouldn't even get to keep our January 20th appointment. Zeki and I had a nice night. It was good to be together.

"In the morning, we went, and here is what we got: 'Shows strong associations with autism spectrum disorder (ASD).' My thought was, we'll go forward. We'll figure it out, we'll get him what he needs. If he has a diagnosis, we can do things with it. I can take it to the school and say, this is what he needs. Because right now—this is what I was thinking then—he's not learning. He spends just as much time in the principal's office as he does in class, and when he's in class, he's not learning. He doesn't go to the principal's office because he's sent there. He goes because he is frustrated, and he knows he can calm down there. He comes home, and he says to me, 'They're all driving me crazy!' He picks up the way other people talk. I say, 'They drive you crazy? Say, frustrated. Say, they make me frustrated.'

"The most important thing for me was, get him to where he can learn in school. I knew something was wrong. I knew that the way they teach wasn't working for him. But the process was terrible. I can hardly tell you because I feel completely blank. Poor Zeki. He was practically throwing up, he was exhausted. He had to leave the assessment halfway through and throw up. He was too nervous to eat. It was nonstop. Do this, do that. He knew he was being tested, but he had no clue if he was doing good or bad. He was constantly under evaluation. For four hours, he was under evaluation. And, you know, I was under evaluation, too! I was thinking, what about parents who are new to the culture? I can speak in English. I've written research papers in English, but what about others?

"I annoyed them a little, I think, because I asked so many questions. I asked questions they couldn't answer. I kept asking, why are you doing this? What does this show? They would be like, tell me animals in the zoo, and he would have to list all the animals in the zoo he could think of. Then he had to jump on one foot. Then he had to trot like a pony. Then they would want him to match things. And it all had to be fast. And if he did poorly on something, he would have to do it again, but he wouldn't want to do it again because he knew he did not do well on it. He hated it, he was feeling like puking. I asked, why are you doing this? What does this task test? No one could say.

"But that's how I always am. I don't give them any reason—I have to be ahead on everything. I'm jumping ahead now. He got the diagnosis, right? I said, OK, we're going to make the best of it. I'm going to use it to make his teachers help him more. I don't give anyone any reason to give up on Zeki. Just the other week, I found out—Zeki isn't allowed to go to recess if it is 30 degrees or colder because of his asthma—and I found out that instead of going to recess, you know where they were putting him? They were putting him in the nurse's office. You know who else is in the nurse's office with him? All the sick kids waiting to be picked up by their parents. When I found that out, my eyes got so big. And I have big eyes! So I had to go to the school.

"I said, 'So, we're keeping him in from recess to reduce the risk of him getting a bacterial infection because he's susceptible from asthma, and, instead, you're putting him in the nurse's office with all the sick kids? Do you see a problem here?'

"They were like, they didn't know what to say. It's like, you have to be there. You have to be on top of everything, meeting the teachers, going to the morning breakfasts, I never miss anything. Now, this one teacher, she emails me every day: 'Zeki wouldn't sit down today. Zeki wouldn't cooperate with another student today. Zeki wouldn't write today.' I'm like, you know I live with him, right? This isn't a surprise to me. But I write back, 'Thank you so much for letting me know. I apologize for this behavior.' And inside, I'm thinking, What the eff! Like, I don't need you to inform me of every little thing he does. Let's talk about solutions. How can he learn? He's good at things, like he's good at math. His math class is the first one, right after his therapy, and I rush him to school, so he won't miss a moment of math, because he's good at it.

"What I was thinking after [the assessment], I was thinking, if he has an autism diagnosis, I can tell that teacher. I can go up to her and say, OK, let's stop describing everything that is wrong. Let's work on solutions. In my job, it's all about solutions. I meet people with no housing, with disabilities, with all kinds of problems. We can't just talk about the problems. It has to be about moving toward solutions. I tell the same thing to Zeki. I tell my son, 'So what? You have autism? OK, that's done. Now: What are you going to do about it? You're not going to sit here and say, I have autism.' And we work together. Now that he has autism, I work with the therapists, speech therapist, occupational therapist, pediatrician. I work with the teachers. I think about parents who can't communicate with the school. My heart goes out to them."

2. The Home Visit

"The assessor[1] visit was the last straw for me. I have blacked the whole thing out. It was a Thursday night; we were coming home from school. I had to pick them up after school. This school—in the winter, it's mayhem. Their school is in our backyard, but they're too close for bussing. In the winter, they can't walk, because they don't plow the alleys. The alleys are the only way to get there because otherwise, it's the highway. So I have to drop them at school, and then I go on my 'lunch break' at 2:15 p.m., but that's really just zooming home to pick them up. If we could get bus service, that would solve it, but we live too close to get the service. For everything there's a rule, and almost every rule is a challenge.

"I was in a frenzy. Zeki had had a bad day at school, he had hit his teacher in the boob. That's a whole different story. He was sent to sit by himself in the nurse's office. He was mad because he didn't want to take off his jacket, but the seatbelt was too tight with his jacket. We had to pick up the baby, who was crying. Even Zakia was upset. The assessor knocks, and there are all our muddy shoes on the walkway. Zeki is in a rage because the baby touched his school bag. Zeki asked the baby nicely, 'Please don't touch my bag.' But the baby kept touching it—of course he did, he's a baby! But Zeki doesn't understand that. He says, 'I did what you said, I asked nicely!' And he hits the baby, yanks his little, short hairs. I grab the baby and take him upstairs because I know Zeki can go in a rage. Zeki is so mad that he pees on himself! Right there in front of the assessor. Then Zakia goes outside without her jacket, and our house is right on the highway. I know Zakia will just get a breath, but this caseworker doesn't know that.

"What is she doing the whole time I'm holding the baby with one hand and using paper towels to mop up Zeki's pee with the other and Zeki's trying to hit the baby? She's sitting on the couch, on my couch, not saying a word and taking notes and wearing her badge like a necklace.

"Next, she has this list of questions. Tell me about Zeki's behavioral issues. Tell me about how he helps around the house. Tell me about his vocabulary. I'm running around, getting snacks, cleaning pee. She can see I'm the only adult here! Not including her. When she left, I told Zakia, we're done.

---

1. One of the first steps to secure a waiver involves a state assessor coming to the applicant's home and submitting a report that verifies the parent's own description of their child with disability. The service is also intended to note needs that the applicant had not already identified; the aim of the assessment is both to verify and help. Usually, the assessment begins with a conversation in which the assessor asks the parent or guardian and, if possible, the child about their daily lives. Then, the assessor observes for around 90 minutes. Nasra's experience didn't align with this format.

"Part of my story, I was thinking about how to fit this in; after that visit, I thought of my husband, and so I'll tell you the story here. He went back to Africa. He couldn't take it. He didn't believe anything was wrong with his son. He still doesn't. It was impossible.

"I said to him, 'Look at the official assessment letter. It says Zeki has ASD and ADHD.' I said to him, 'Here it is, how can you deny this?'

"He said, 'It's not true. It's the government. The government wants him to have that diagnosis. They can control him and track him that way. They can track us.'

"I said, 'Would they give him this diagnosis if it wasn't true? This diagnosis means that we can apply for things, for grants, for money. They don't want to give families a diagnosis, because then they have to give families money!'

"He says it's more important to them to control families. He says Zeki is fine, and that the government is lying to us and trying to make us believe Zeki is sick.

"How can I communicate with that? Even though it's just me, I know that it is better for all of us that he left. I hadn't felt so alone as when the assessor was over in a long time. It's how I felt when we would be screaming at each other. Now he's back in Africa. I don't want anything from him. I keep pictures of us in our home for the kids. Zakia talks to him sometimes. If it wasn't for them, I wouldn't have anything to do with him. He still calls me to say there is nothing wrong with Zeki, that everything I'm doing for him—all the research, the doctors, there are so many doctors, you should see all the doctors we see, the therapy—that every single thing I'm doing, how I've turned my life upside down, is for nothing, for a lie.

"I thought of those words when the assessor left. I didn't think the government was watching us. It was the opposite. They didn't care."

3. The Naturopath

Ally and I pulled up in our cars outside Nasra's townhome at the same time. It was also the same time as Nasra's two older children, Zeki and Zakia, were returning from Duxy, an after-school program held at their mosque. Ally greeted Zeki cheerfully, and he didn't acknowledge her. He grabbed his tablet and sat in the far corner of the room. Ally was unphased; she asked Zakia a few questions about assignments she was working on at school, and then played with Hassan while Nasra set out one bowl of grapes and a second bowl of sliced cucumbers. Zakia went upstairs to work on her homework, and Nasra and Ally looked over Nasra's food log, in which she noted all the food Zeki had eaten in one column and summarized each day's ups and downs in the next column. The two women discussed Zeki's diet—what seemed to be working, what could be adjusted, what might be worth eliminating—while playing with the baby and feeding him ripped up cucumbers. After going through the food diary, they agreed that the probiotic chewables were calming Zeki's indigestion. They remained concerned about his struggles in school—reports of hitting teachers, tangling with classmates, and getting sent out of the class.

"He's not going to learn," Nasra sighed.

Ally showed Nasra a set of brochures for a specialized probiotic company; she wondered whether probiotics attuned to Zeki's microbiome could continue to help with his gastrointestinal issues while also improving his mood and attention.

"You send in a stool sample every four months, and they adjust, so it keeps up with him as he's changing," Ally explained. "They send a report with each customization, so that we can make sure everything's working in sync and nothing's canceling something else out."

They talked about cost, and Nasra stressed that she needed a new job soon. "I need something more," she told Ally, "Something with a big company, a big organization, a large employer. I just need something solid with a big company. Kids are, like, money—toothbrush, toothpaste, everything costs money."

"I know," Ally said. "I'm going to talk to my friend at [a large medical device company]. I didn't see her this week, but I'm seeing her next weekend."

"Thank you," Nasra said. "I'm working on my resume, making sure everything is perfect."

"Oh!" Ally stood up to grab her bag in the kitchen. "I brought you the oil sample. It's the only sample I could get, but if you like it, we'll see what we can do." Ally handed a sleek pump bottle to Nasra, who read the label closely.

"This is the . . ." Nasra began.

Ally cut in, "It's not an active ingredient."

Nasra laughed, handed me the bottle, and explained, "It's so natural that it's from marijuana, can you believe it?"

Ally tried to offer a longer explanation, but Nasra kept speaking: "It doesn't have the THC, that's what Ally keeps telling me. It's just hemp, there's no drugs. Well," Nasra shrugged elaborately, "it is natural, right?"

"Do you want to try the evening one now?" Ally asked.

Both women looked over at Zeki, who was absorbed in his tablet, and Ally voiced the thought that seemed to be shared between them: "You can do it after bath tonight, it's easy. Text me. Tell me how he responds at bedtime."

I asked Ally and Nasra what they hoped the oil would do, and Nasra had a ready explanation. "My biggest thing," Nasra began,

I just need to get him to regulate his internal reactions. That's my number one goal: self-regulation. When he feels an emotion, I have to teach him how to respond to it. Autism, it means children will feel emotions so intensely, at the slightest thing. The Internet is slow? And it makes him feel enraged? He has to learn to recognize that feeling and respond, walk away into a room, get himself alone. Because right now, he can't do that. He sees things—like the baby, he doesn't recognize the baby is a baby. The baby drools on him, and he is trying to throw the baby down the stairs. I can't go to the bathroom without bringing one of them into the bathroom with me. I cannot leave them in a room together without me. You see? The oil, it gives a feeling of well-being. And that will help him reflect, think, articulate. It detoxifies him.

"It's an herbal remedy," Ally told me. "The herbs come from the foothills in Burma. It can detoxify the body from heavy metals."

After the exchange of the oil, Ally stayed over for a little while longer. She and Nasra talked about school, and Nasra let Ally read Zeki's latest treatment reports. Ally wrote down a list of questions that she thought Nasra should raise with Zeki's therapists. Hassan started leaving us and trying to tap on Zeki's tablet, but Zeki played with the baby and didn't get upset.

"I see what he can be," Nasra told us. Ally nodded.

Five Topoi across Microbiome Stories

After departing the WCAG, Nasra, as well as Layla, Farah, Asma, and Asha, turned to the human microbiome to understand autism.[2] This section maps how participating mothers found in the microbiome an epistemology and related care practices that meshed with their daily lives and beliefs. This section is organized by five topoi,[3] or general categories from which participating mothers made claims about the body, disability, caregiving, and health. These

---

2. Participants' adoptions of microbiome care were not anomalies. Decoteau (2021) has documented how Somali mothers in Toronto built an "epistemic community" grounded in a shared understanding of autism as caused by microbiological imbalances wrought by migration to North America. In Toronto, Somali mothers collaborated with university scientists to investigate microbiome and autism connections and, specifically, to study how configurations of gut bacteria among Somali refugees might contribute to autism (pp. 182–187).

3. The rhetorical term *topoi* refers to commonplace topics from which people might make arguments (or, in this case, form health beliefs). In classical rhetoric, Aristotle identified topoi as general categories, shared by rhetors and audiences and from which rhetors could build arguments; topoi thus enable rhetors to start with broad categories, or commonplaces, and then develop specific content and arguments from these categories.

topoi are not necessarily commonplaces from which rhetors compose spoken or written arguments. These topoi are commonplaces from which rhetors advance rhetorical refusal. As I have argued throughout this book, rhetorical refusal is a communicative, meaning-making, disruptive, participatory act, but one that is not necessarily enacted through the traditional rhetorical modes, speaking or writing to an audience. Accordingly, these topoi recognize commonplaces that are often material, practice-based sites from which rhetors shape rhetorical refusal. These topoi mark the sites at which health epistemologies and discourses became, for participating mothers, real—concrete, material, actionable. At these sites, rhetors opted in or opted out, they made mistakes, remained silent, leveraged wrong vocabularies, adopted experimental care practices, rejected medical advice, folded up a form and left it in their car, or walked away. These topoi build a rhetorical framework useful to listen to medical dissent as rhetorical refusal, a framework I explain at the end of this chapter.

Topos 1—Medicine

Nasra, Layla, Farah, Asma, and Asha practiced microbiome-informed caregiving that relied on accessible medicines such as food, time spent outside, sun exposure, infused creams and oils, and interactions with animals. These nonspecialized tools extended agency to parents in a child's healthcare. By contrast, when I talked to participating mothers about mainstream medical care, mothers commonly spoke about pills they didn't like, scripts they could not decipher, and therapies they did not understand. Nasra, in her narrative, positioned Zeki's autism screening as a pivotal point at which she turned from medical care; Nasra described being relegated to the sidelines while an inscrutable autism screening unfolded. Farah, in a focus group interview, reported that she did not take her son to an autism screening that his school had recommended for several years, because, Farah told the small group, "I don't want to take my child to the doctor and get pills. It's the ADHD pills that worry me. Doctors only give you pills" (2/17/2018). Another Somali American mother, Ayaan, urged Farah to reconsider and explained, "You don't have to take pills if you take him for a screening. They just give you information." But Farah was convinced that any interaction with medicine would set her on a pharmaceutical path of which she would lose control. She responded to Ayaan, "But he's very hyper. He's like my neighbor's child, who is sick and has pills. But [my son] is younger. The last time I went to the doctor? She wanted me to take pills. I said, I cannot take pills every day. I am not a machine, I'm a human" (2/17/2018). Another mother averred that the school and therapists were always pushing prescription medications on her son, and the fourth participant said that her daughter had turned into a "zombie" on prescription medication (2/17/2018). These mothers saw healthcare as a system that prescribed their children personality-altering drugs, drugs that they had no path toward understanding.

Mothers' stories about microbiome care were different, and one key difference was that microbial medicines were everyday foods, lotions, and environmental changes, procured and administered by parents themselves. Pollan (2013) unpacked the DIY accessibility of microbial medicines for the *New York Times Magazine* when he wrote that "the outlines of a diet for the new superorganism were coming clear, and it didn't require the ministrations of the food scientists at Nestlé or General Mills to design it. [. . .] The components of a microbiota-friendly diet are already on the supermarket shelves and in farmers' markets." Indeed, all five participating Somali mothers used diet as their primary medicine. Even as the food items used to rebalance a child's microbiome became more specialized and harder to find—yogurt with specific cultures, almond-flour crackers, chia seeds—these items were still procurable by mothers themselves. No doctors' appointments or scripts required. Farah described how her diet interventions worked: "[My son] is a picky eater. The first thing I did, before I knew much, I took out all the sugar. He used to just scream, out of nowhere, and that stopped. He would listen to me. Take out sugar, and he changed. Then I started working on carbohydrates" (2/20/2019). Using microbiome-informed care, Farah could change her son's diet and then directly observe how these interventions affected her child. In Farah's story, parents were less consumers of medicine than they were collaborative producers of health knowledge and situated caregiving. Nasra also used diet as a primary medicine in her son's microbiome care; Nasra showed me a chart that her oldest daughter, Zakia, had made for Zeki; on the sheet of loose-leaf paper, Zakia had drawn all the foods that her younger brother was now encouraged to eat—broccoli, zucchini, salmon, almonds, dates, and chicken. All the food items were smiling. On the flip side, she had drawn food that he wasn't supposed to eat—chips, cookies, bread, milk—with *x*'s across them. The diet had become a family affair, a mode of expertise and form of caregiving that children and parents understood and practiced together.

In my first post-WCAG interview with Farah, she explained how she used probiotics as medicine to help her son's microbiome:

> I use probiotics. Do you know what those are? You can get probiotic pills at the grocery store. I'll show you mine. The thing to look for is how many

colonies there are. Bacteria colonies. Because you want more colonies. Does that make sense? You need to get more bacteria into the microbiome so it's healthier. I go to a store and buy my own. We're using them every day, and [my son's] having less stomach issues. Now I'm looking at the diet, too; it's all connected. So, if he eats less bread and just all the processed food here, then that will help his bacteria, too. (12/5/2018)

I had first met Farah a few months earlier when she had been a participant in the WCAG program; like many parents, Farah had delegated the writing of her application to a community health worker and left the program when her proposed plan was denied funding. Now, Farah was working at home with a naturopath and was teaching me about the microbiome and explaining how she translated microbiome understandings of human health into specific interventions for her family.

Most WCAG participants had assumed a similar role to Farah's. As described in chapter 3, Khadija had brought to Midnimo a plastic bag filled with medical communications—bills, reports, vaccination records, annual health assessments, appointment reminders, holiday cards from pediatric clinics, and scripts. This bag stood in for her own account of her children and their health. Mothers often told me that they wanted "medical papers" for their children. Participants recognized that they needed papers to gain resources, but built into the term *papers* was a concession that they, the parents, would not understand their contents and would only use them for their exchange value. Microbial theories of autism did not function as vast networks of specialized knowledge that parents needed but could not access. Farah's etiology illustrates how participating parents positioned themselves as experts within microbiome-informed healthcare routines. In these routines, parents like Farah acquired, controlled, understood, evaluated, and adjusted all medications, which were primarily food and nutritional supplements and creams. Anchored in everyday medicines, microbial theories of autism offered an accessible body of knowledge, strands of which parents could braid into their lives and vernaculars.

Topos 2—Location

Participating mothers enacted microbiome care at home. Nasra's story depicts some implications of a shift of care from clinic to home. Nasra began her story with her laborious journey to get her son assessed for autism. They sat on a wait list for months. She sprung for a motel because she was worried that driving to the appointment would be too risky; they might have been late, and the center would have already moved on to the next appointment. During the assessment, Zeki and Nasra were hungry and tired. Nasra handed her son over to a form of professional scrutiny that she felt obligated to use but that she could not begin to explain or trust. This unease did not end after the assessment. An autism diagnosis sent Nasra and Zeki into a spiral of specialist appointments. Nasra scheduled speech therapy for Zeki in the dark hours before school, occupational therapy after school. For participants like Nasra, the medical world was a separate, disorienting world. Parents shuttled children to rigidly scheduled doctors' appointments, therapists' appointments, and assessments. Then parents took children back to their other world, the one with family, home, grocery shopping, neighbors, a language they knew. The two worlds were brightly divided, incommensurate.

The experience of home care was different. With naturopaths who came to their home, parents got time back in their days. The stress of arriving at appointments on time evaporated. The pressure of having to get a child ready or many children ready—snacks packed, toys packed, diapers and wipes, water bottles filled—for a doctor's was alleviated. Convenience, however, was only one dimension of how at-home appointments shifted the autism experience. Mothers collaborated with their naturopaths to analyze a child's body and behaviors and to chart a plan. In contrast to Nasra's experience with a county assessor visiting her home, a naturopath came to a family's home to deliver care. In Nasra's living room, Nasra and Ally spent the evening going over Nasra's food diary and making sense of how Zeki's food correlated with his behaviors that week. Together, they were connecting the dots into a coherent shape.

Rhetoricians have shown how the material spaces in which healthcare unfolds—hospital, clinic, home, nonmedical facility, university—not only shape patient experience but also allow different types of knowledge to gain traction. Specialized medical knowledge reigns in institutional spaces of medicine, while embodied knowledge "becomes suspect, if not dismissible, when read through the lens of technological, scientific knowledge" (Owens, 2013, p. 251). As discussed in this book's introduction, in spaces of institutional medicine, those who speak from the vantage point of medicine and scientific evidence speak with epistemic privilege of being "knowers," or "experts whose judgment and knowledge count" (Lay, 2000, p. 22), while others speak from a position of "epistemic marginalization" (Fricker, 2007). But in spaces intentionally carved outside of the hospital's walls, a patient's own vernaculars, suspicions, and lived knowledge, typically "evidence appropriate in that private sphere," gain credibility (Schuster, 2006, p. 10). Historians and scholars of childbirth have shown how, as childbirth moved from the home to the hospital in the mid-twentieth century, the practices of lay midwifery and generational experiential knowledge about childbirth were drained of credibility and expertise, and childbirth became the purview of male, medical doctors (Leavitt, 1986; Lay, 2000). Microbiome at-home care could be seen as reversing this consolidation of expertise. Microbial etiologies of autism allowed for a relocation of caregiving to the home and, in doing so, materialized expertise, care, and control differently. Mothers could voice experiential knowledge and have their stories and perspectives taken seriously to make health decisions. Appointments with naturopaths recoded the home as a space of both care and knowledge production.

Topos 3—Affect

Participating mothers often described microbiome care as having a positive, affective dimension, separate from its purported therapeutic usefulness. Microbiome care practices were not just a means to an end, but the practices themselves were enjoyable for whole families. Nasra described how Zakia enjoyed drawing her brother's diet plans. Nasra also described how she, her naturopath, and her children enjoyed snacks together in the family room. Farah spoke to this dimension when she told a story about goat therapy, suggested by a friend and endorsed by Farah's naturopath as a means to repopulate her son's microbiome. Farah narrated her family's experience:

> A parent told me about it [goat therapy]. We're trying it. That's what we do: try everything. What we do is we go to one of those white German Minnesota farms. The first time they saw us, we were not the family they were expecting! I felt like we were in a movie. But it makes sense for us Somalis. We're not used to the medicine and environment in the US. You have everything indoors, processed, medicine for everything, birth control, the vaccines, the food. For the microbiome, they have these germ-free mice they do experiments with. It's very interesting. The mice show that the body can't adapt to everything being processed. It's time we get back outside with animals. When the children play with goats, their bodies grow stronger, they start to develop healthy bacteria. My son, he likes the goats. He has fun there! It's so different from therapy, where it's "do this, no you're doing it wrong, no you can't do that." (12/20/2018)

Farah first explained that she had done her due diligence—she had read about microbiome theories of autism and mice experiments, and the explanations had made sense to her and had aligned with her experience. Farah offered a medical rationale for goat therapy but then noted that goat therapy was fun. The whole time Farah told this story, she was smiling, and her tone was lively. Goat therapy brought her family together. Goat therapy was valuable not only for the progress it promised but in and of itself. It was time well spent.

Farah's description of goat therapy stood in contrast to Nasra's desolate description of her son wilting during his daylong autism screening. Farah's story also stood in contrast to the ways that the WCAG sought to label children by their deficits. In WCAG grant-writing sessions and Midnimo health literacy classes, Somali mothers reiterated that they wanted rhetorical space to talk about their children as children—loved, complex, indelible individuals, not as columns of burdens and strengths, deficits and goals. But they instead encountered state forms asking them to list the ways that their children burdened their families, assessors with notepads and credentials, and charts with prescribed goals. The microbiome, by contrast, offered parents and children space to be themselves and to engage in therapeutic activities that brought out their best selves. Playing with goats, eating together, drawing smiling almonds—in these activities, children were not evaluated and scored; in these activities, children shone as themselves. There was an affective dimension to microbiome care that worked in a way that was not dependent on its therapeutic effectiveness. Farah's goat story suggests that microbiome-focused care was preferable not only because the materials were accessible and did not require trips to the doctor's office as well as disorienting bouts of surveillance, scripts, and insurance codes; microbiome care was also preferable because it felt good. Care involved preparing food alongside family members; care involved eating grapes with a naturopath and recounting positive moments in the last week; care involved loading up into a car and going to a goat farm.

Importantly, positive, affective care experiences were not limited to naturopathic microbiome care. One mother, Saidiyo, told me that after she was rejected from the WCAG program, she went to a pediatrician who specialized in autism and whom a friend had recommended. Saidiyo reported that she had had a great experience, and she was now committed to continuing to work with this provider. What was different? Saidiyo described the practice and why she was won over:

> Do you know Michelle and Heather? They have a clinic, and they work with autistic kids. Almost everyone there has kids with autism, all the nurses and the doctors. One nurse had four of her own kids with autism. They all have some connection. When you go there, in the waiting room, there are all these mismatched chairs, it is so nice. It feels like home. I get there, and I feel [that] I am at home. I can relax. The lobby is cozy and has mismatched

chairs and a fireplace. It's the kind of place where you can just relax. They ask you how you are doing, and they know how it is. The waiting room, I keep talking about the waiting room because that's how the whole place is. The waiting room is just so cozy. You can sit by a fireplace. [. . .] It's just *nice*. It's just like home. Like, come here and relax. It doesn't feel clinical. It doesn't feel cold. It doesn't feel like you're at the doctor's. (2/2/2018)

Saidiyo used the words *nice, relaxing,* and *home* to describe her experience at the new clinic. She referred to the two pediatricians by their first names and explained that the providers had personal experiences raising autistic children and that they shared these experiences with their patients. What was the clinical examination like? What did the doctors prescribe? What were the next steps? Saidiyo addressed none of these questions in her story. The important parts were affect and relationships. She had found a place where she and her children felt safe and calm. She now had a trusted healthcare provider.

Farah's goat therapy story and Saidiyo's pediatrician story depict that the affective, relational side of healthcare is not only important but pivotal. The affective experience can shape whether a parent entrusts a child's healthcare with a microbiome-informed naturopath or an allopathic pediatrician. Saidiyo, Nasra, and Farah all spoke to how, often, medical spaces felt cold and alienating, and prior chapters have shown that Somali parents experienced medical discourses of autism as deficit-based and stifling. Again and again, parents described the growing awareness that "healthcare does not (finally) make space for us, its patients. Instead, it alters daily practices in ways that do not necessarily fit well with the intricacies of our diseases" (Mol, 2008, p. 2)—or, I would add, our health. For some parents, microbiome care was a relational opting out—an opting out of cold waiting rooms, clinics that felt like clinics, inscrutable providers who parents saw twice a year, specialists who did not directly engage parents, and the checklists of all of a child's deficits. They were opting into a feeling, into a healthcare experience that left a positive affective residue, that felt good, that made a child happy, that brought a family together.

Topos 4—Story

As described earlier in this chapter, the human microbiome is individualized and enmeshed in constant interplay with its environment. Microbiome composition reflects an individual's history, environment, diet, moves, pets, cohabitating humans, occupations, and more (Pollan, 2013; Yong, 2016; Rees and Gilman, 2018). If the composition of the human microbiome is a result of lived experiences and exposures, then one's personal history is critical clinical information. Microbiologist Emma Allen-Vercoe has envisioned that new "microbial ecosystem therapeutics" might address chronic diseases that are currently poorly treated, and that such therapeutics would be "tailored to a given patient's lifestyle and gut microbiota individuality" (2013, p. 628). For Somali American participants, the microbiome's emphasis on personal history meant that experiences of forced migration, loss, trauma, resettlement, and daily stress left clinically significant marks on their children's health.

In microbiome care, naturopaths not only elicited a patient's or caregiver's story but used that story as a foundation for care. Nasra's account illustrates the disheartening experience of failing to tell one's story to a consequential audience. First, Nasra brought her son to an assessment center, where she and her son could respond only to the questions asked directly of them, questions for which Nasra could not decipher the motivating logic. Nasra then described the experience of having an assessor arrive at her home to document Nasra's family life. Nasra thought of the broader context and smaller moments that the assessor would never know because she would not ask. The only story that mattered—the story that would stand in for Zeki's family life in his application—was the scene, a hectic one at the end of a long school day, that the assessor watched unfold. Another mother, Sofia, said of a report that an assessor had written about her son: "I'm sure it all happened just the way she wrote it. But when I read it, I feel sick to my stomach. It feels so cold" (3/1/2018). Home visits left Nasra and Sofia feeling alone. Although they were being watched, they felt unseen. Both mothers described feeling like their stories were disappearing beneath the accounts of uninvested, cold observers. By beginning microbiome care, Nasra was also refusing the stories that medical and state experts told about her family. Nasra's experience of voicelessness changed with the microbiome. Here, parents like Nasra found joint rhetorical and clinical tools with which to tell their stories and make convincing arguments that their distinct embodied histories marked their bodies in ways that merited distinct care.

Participating Somali American mothers were not alone in seeking alternatives to evidence-based medicine and its reliance on population evidence. Writing about the appeal of alternative healthcare, rhetorician Colleen Derkatch (2016) has described why randomized control trials, the gold standard of medical evidence, can nonetheless repel potential patients. Writes Derkatch:

> The numbers produced in biomedical research are emptied of their social interest through their method of production, the randomized controlled

trial, which transforms a variable range of health problems, treatments, practitioners, and patients into measurable phenomena by operating within rigid criteria and practices. This transformation of people, practices, and effects into measurable phenomena allows us to compare "disparate objects" according to a shared metric. (p. 32)

It was these numbers emptied of bodies, experiences, concerns, histories, and social interests that Somali participants also rejected. Such socially cleansed evidence, participants have argued, was harmful to those whose aberrant social histories might matter to their health and receptivity to medicine. In chapter 2, Somali parents considered that while American-administered vaccines might be fine for most children, that didn't mean that these vaccines were fine for all children, especially Somali American children whose backgrounds and somatic experiences were not represented in clinical trials or in the experiences of the majority. When it came to vaccines, Somali American parents did not find a rhetorical platform with which to make effectual arguments about their concerns. If expressed in public discourse, their concerns were often misheard as symptoms of scientific illiteracy and signs of antivaccination infiltration. But the microbiome offered a scientific discourse with which to advance these arguments. All five microbiome-ascribing Somali mothers cited migration and its aftermath as reasons for autism. Asha, Nasra, and Farah explained that their children's microbiota were better suited to sub-Saharan climates than Northern ones. Asha and Layla explained that an influx of antibiotics imperiled their children's microbiota. All five participants cited Western diets—processed foods, too many carbs, an overload of preservatives—as a source of autism. When I asked Asha about her understanding of autism, she explained, "I always knew that something had changed when we came here. So, when [the naturopath] said, well, your children's gut fits Africa. It's going to struggle here in Minnesota. That was what I felt" (6/22/2018). Microbiome care welcomed parents to tell their stories, have these stories matter in a clinically relevant way, and build care responsive to experiences of displacement, resettlement, and structural precarity.

In a final example of the power of personal story within microbiome care, Asma used the microbiome as a framework that not only explained her daughter Fatha's autism as a consequence of forced migration but that specifically grounded Fatha's autism in her family's personal experiences of loss. Asma explained:

When we came here, both of my children were young, and they got a lot of vaccinations. I don't remember, maybe I should have paid more attention. Then, Fatha had cellulitis, and she was on antibiotics. Antibiotics can affect her microbes. Then, when we came here, they ate very differently. One thing, I've heard I'm not the only one, but when we came here, we bought a lot of canned food, and we were eating food for cats. Why would you sell animal and human food in the same store? I still think that. It is an awful time, when you first come here, with two children. We were staying in a place that always smelled bad, it wasn't nice, so I don't know if there was a cause there. The water was brown, the air was bad, and no one would do anything about it. Cat food also could affect the microbes.

This whole time, their father is not here. He's in Africa. So, everything is not right. She never spoke. Since we came to America, she has not said one real word. Audrey [Asma's friend from their children's shared public school, who introduced Asma to microbiome-driven theories of autism] said things like school, the Purell, being inside, all can cause autism. That wasn't how life was in Africa.

To describe her understanding of autism as caused by microbiome dysbiosis, Asma spoke about specific and searing experiences shouldered by her family: a child's bout with cellulitis; a family far from home; an unlivable apartment and unbothered landlord; a father kept from his family by an ocean and refugee quotas. Asma then drew from a microbial, clinical discourse to frame her longtime understanding of bodies and illness in both scientific validity and meaningful plot. Rhetorically, Asma used the microbiome to somaticize loss. Lost family members and lost traditions materialized in the extinction of microbial species. The realization she had been feeding her children cat food did not just dissolve into general anxiety but could be pinpointed in a colony of new bacteria. The experience of making unheard complaint after unheard complaint about brown tap water to a landlord became narratively enfolded into the coating of a child's intestines.

For other participants, the suspicions, for example, that "our kids don't get enough sun. It's cold, and they're inside a lot. Some people say the weather is too hard on their bodies" (Layla, 5/12/2018) or that "[our children] are exposed to toxins every day, and mothers know it's making their kids sick, but there's nothing to do about it" (Farhiyo, 3/19/2018) or that "our bodies weren't meant for this place" (Farhiyo, 3/19/2018) were no longer dismissible musings but were statements that could be linked up to physical evidence—missing microbes and their symptoms. On their own, these suspicions were roving and imprecise, a felt sense that something was not right. But in the microbiome framework, these residues, these gut feelings, these emotional intensities, these unsayable memories slotted into scientific frameworks and systems of evidence. Stories of loss, alienation, and discrimination became differently real when tied to somatic referents. Past life experiences became traceable effects on a child's body. The past was no longer just something that happened, irrevocable and oftentimes unspeakable. The past materialized into the present as actionable clinical evidence. Microbial explanations and treatments of autism offered parents medically innovative ways to reinvest these numbers, bodies, symptoms, and etiologies with social meaning (Derkatch, 2016)—with their own stories.

Having a space to tell their stories and have these stories matter in their children's healthcare also extended control to parents; in prior chapters, parents held back from engaging with healthcare, including from vaccinating their children, because they feared that doing so would slot them into a system that demanded their compliance but offered no safety net should something go wrong. Within the microbiome, parents enjoyed a firmer sense of control, in part because the microbiome was not an abstract system of knowledge but an accessible etiology that could be infused with one's own personal history and envisioned future. Writing about the political and ethical dimensions of telling stories, Yam (2019) has explained that storytelling "stem[s] from the almost universal human desire to render events coherent so that one can grapple with the ongoing uncertainties and contingencies of life" and that "the telling of one's stories, therefore, provides a rhetorical platform for interlocutors to explore their relationships with one another and with the uncontrollable forces in their lives" (p. 39). The microbiome as a health-explanatory framework offered a theory for the relationships between large-scale world events and systems, the personal experience of these events and systems, and individual bodies. The microbiome proved pliable to explain otherwise "uncontrollable forces in their [our] lives" (Yam, 2019, p. 39). The microbiome offered a practical handbook for gaining (or feeling like one was gaining) some control within deleterious systems. Using microbiome-informed therapeutics, mothers could exert some control over how these complex systems manifested in their family life and their bodies. Control came through connecting experiences big and small, experiences that often made their havers feel like they were at the mercy of large, uncontrollable systems and relations. Mothers could bring together forced migration, cat food consumption, embodied behaviors, family separation, impossibly expensive produce, unlawful evictions, bullying at school, a new diagnosis, and longing for home together into one plot. In turn, mothers could treat embodied symptoms of the past and of complex geopolitical forces through diet, time outdoors, sunshine, and probiotics. The microbiome provides a frame wherein stories have not only narrative meaning but somatic significance, where telling a story can not only bring a meaningful plot to a life but can also unlock clinically significant knowledge and correspond with a course of care.

Topos 5—Social Determinants of Health

Microbiome discourses of autism offered not only a form of healthcare in which individual story mattered but also a scientific explanation for how forced migration and resettlement brought unique health problems for refugees. For these reasons, microbiome etiologies of health and illness could be used to center social determinants of health and upstream causes of health disparities and to call for collective action. Specifically, the microbiome provided a framework for responding to autism as a Western illness (Decoteau, 2021)—not a Western illness in the sense that autism only exists in the West but a Western illness in the sense that Western modernity, systemic racism, and conditions of late capitalism have engendered "modern plagues" of chronic conditions (MacFabe, 2013, p. 52) and that refugees might be particularly susceptible (Luzopone et al., 2012; Mulle, Sharp, and Cubells, 2013; Toh and Allen-Vercoe, 2015).

This and the previous chapters have documented stories from participants who read autism as a bodily sign that something was wrong with Western life and that marginalized persons had to shoulder the risks of Western modernity while their affluent and white counterparts enjoyed its fruits. "Mothers know it's making their kids sick," Farhiyo said of life in Minnesota, "but there's nothing to do about it" (3/19/2018). Anab explained, "If you take a huge group of people and suddenly migrate them to a different place, then there are going to be effects and consequences" (4/15/2018). Neither Farhiyo nor Anab spoke about the microbiome, but their explanations for why autism might happen more often in Somali American children could be mapped onto a microbiome etiology of autism. All five mothers who took up microbiome care offered the following definitions of autism as connected to Western, depletive environments:

- Everything is genetic; white or Somali, things in your environment can turn off or awaken different genes. Toxins are not good for anyone, but if your mother and her mother ate GMOs, and you eat GMOs, your body has adapted. For our children, their bodies haven't adapted. —Layla, 9/2/2018
- The connection seems to be autism and antibiotics. Antibiotics kill good bacteria, and in America, kids are always taking antibiotics. Parents have to work, they give their kids antibiotics, kids stop coughing, can go back to school, parents go back to work. We know it's causing big problems. —Nasra, 5/21/2018
- Somalis in Africa, their ecosystem fits in Africa. You bring it here, and it doesn't fit. It's diverse, it's healthy, but it's healthy for Africa. You add the

food, the medicine, the cold. Our microbiomes aren't ready. That's why Somali kids get autism more than, and more severe than, your kids [white kids]. —Asha, 8/10/2018
- It's cold, and they're inside a lot. Too many vaccines, too many antibiotics. Their bodies can't handle it. I bring them in for one problem, and it's, OK, here is a new pill to get, and then it's a new problem. So that is one reason the bacteria make sense. Their bodies are all off because this isn't where we belong. —Asma, 5/12/2018
- The houses we live in are in poor condition. There's mold, dirty air, dirty water. We're nomads, we are meant to move, be outside, get sun, and here we are in houses, crowded, no air, polluted air, dirty, the water comes out dirty. People say it makes kids sick, and the microbiome explains why. Their bacteria are wiped out. —Farah, 5/27/2018

These definitions of autism illustrate a pattern documented in the previous three chapters: participants used the term *autism* to reference community sickness, that is, multiple, intersecting hardships specific to Somalis Americans' experiences of forced migration, resettlement, poverty, and systemic racism.

Community sickness was not a new concept, but it was given new validity by the science-aligned microbiome discourses—as Farah said, "people say it makes kids sick, and the microbiome explains why" (5/27/2018). Microbiome discourses did not only explain autism as a specific experience for Somalis in diaspora, but the microbiome also outlined specific care practices that responded to and sought to heal the lived experience of community sickness, described in chapter 1. If ill health is wrought by inequities built into Western life, treatment should not just attend to bodies, even situated bodies, but should attend to structural causes of Western diseases. The microbiome theory of autism offered a discourse with which Somali American parents could make this argument. Using microbiome discourses, parents could insist upon addressing the questions: What about Western life is unevenly sickening people? What about resettlement in the United States is harming Somali American children? These were the questions that Somali mothers refused to abandon when their health literacy teachers asked them to define autism. These were the questions that Somali American parents were asking when they suggested that vaccines may not be safe for their children. These were the arguments that Somali mothers were making when they tried to tell WCAG administrators that they wanted different, localized care practices, not just adaptive swim lessons. But in medical, public health, and social services, such questions were dismissed as logistically impossible and as signs of Somali parents' scientific, medical, and bureaucratic illiteracy. Autism is a neurodevelopmental disability, Somali parents were told. Vaccines are safe and effective, Somali parents were told. There are rules about using public funds, Somali parents were told. In the microbiome discourses, however, there was rhetorical infrastructure to talk about social determinants of health as causes of community sickness for Somali American families. The microbiome equipped Somali American parents with a discourse to publicly fight for recognition of the uneven, environmental causes of community sickness and to privately care for their families. In microbiome etiologies, autism was a community sickness—and it was treatable as such.

Following Refusal's Arc: The Microbiome's Health Futures

Throughout this book, I have theorized rhetorical refusal as prosocial, affiliative, participatory, and future-oriented. As hopeful. Rhetorical refusals through microbiome care practices are no exception. Here, microbiome care practices are just as much of an opting out of medical relationships, knowledge, and care as they are an opting into an alternative set of knowledges, relationships, stories, and care practices. Somali American mothers' practices of microbiome care were "communion-centered" and "future-oriented," a "promise to one's child of future good health and a vow to one's associates of continual association" (Sobo, 2016, p. 347). Each casein-free snack prepared, goat farm visited, antibiotic declined, microbiome website consulted was a further separation from medicine and an incremental materialization of different etiologies of healthcare, caregiving, knowledge-making, and parenting. Each probiotic-infused lotion applied, each prebiotic regime carried out, each naturopath's phone number passed along was a rhetorical refusal, enacted at the level of everyday routine. These rhetorical refusals do not arc toward abstract futures but participate in on-the-ground future-making, right here, right now. What are the futures that Somali American mothers' acts of microbiome care were building?

First, Somali American mothers' microbiome care practices were building a health future where patients and caregivers were informed collaborators in their healthcare. Lived experiences, family histories, and experiential knowledge were essential to making diagnoses and treatment plans. Second, this health future centered social determinants of health in diagnosis and care. The discourses of the microbiome offered a vocabulary and framework to draw connections between personal and collective histories, life experiences, social structures and inequities, and somatic phenomena. Somali American participants, in turn, operationalized microbiome discourses as a scientific language to name, discuss, and act on structural causes of illness. In chapter 1, I argued that Somali health literacy students rejected medical definitions of autism in part because they bracketed structural causes of health and illness. Medical definitions of autism fell into the pattern of "science [having] a tendency to ignore the fact that cultural, structural, and ideological conditions have also carved up the world, rendering particular populations vulnerable to poor health conditions, lower life expectancies, and higher levels of distrust and discrimination" (Decoteau, 2021, p. 216). Parents found in the microbiome rhetorical and scientific tools useful to cohere this carved-up world, to center social determinants of health and upstream sources of health disparities in their healthcare. This shift from a neurodevelopmental model of autism to a microbiome model of autism was a movement away from a specialized and individualized approach to illness to a structural and environmental understanding of illness, what Happe (2013) has called an ecosocial model of care.

Third, if autism is framed as caused by structural and historical conditions that somaticize at the level of the individual body, then the appropriate course of action is not more of the same—early diagnoses, state grants, state-funded therapies, "individualized educational plans." The appropriate course of action is to live differently and to fight for structural change so that people *can* live differently. Eat real foods, be outside, travel. At the structural level: eliminate food deserts, scrutinize medical interventions, address poor air quality and housing environments, and research the understudied health effects of migration. The microbiome equipped participating parents with a set of scientific-adjacent discourses useful to publicly fight for recognition of environmental health risks—community sickness—and to privately care for their families outside of medical and state evaluation and intervention.

Fourth, microbiome etiologies of autism arced toward a health future where health publics were biosocial health collectives that formed on the shared lived experiences of illness. In the beginning of this study, when the WCAG workshops were getting started, I watched new participants gather at Midnimo because they identified as parents of children who were sick. But, as described in chapter 3, as I watched each mother work with a community health worker, I also watched this group disband. The disability services application process revised the category "sick children" into diagnostic categories and subcategories. Mothers who did not secure WCAG funding left Midnimo not only without grant funds but also without the support of prior, informal parent networks. However, following the five participants whose stories inform this chapter, I watched this fragmentation occur in reverse. Mothers reclaimed autism as a diffuse somatic experience. Mothers used the microbiome rhetorically to broaden autism back into community sickness. Inclusion in microbiome-informed autism communities was based not on a shared diagnosis but on shared social experiences of illness. Autism was not a private, medical matter managed by doctors and therapists but a lodestone to gather parents navigating community sickness. In microbiome-informed autism-as-community-sickness communities, Khadija would be included; her experiences of caring for her children's mysterious illness, of advocating for her children at school, and of vying for help in an unfeeling healthcare system would be validated. Sofia and her son would be included, with or without a SMRT diagnosis. Ayan's explanations for why she needed a tented bed and stroller would be readily understood. The WCAG parents envisioning care through return migrations, housing stability, and diet overhauls would be enfolded without having to justify their inclusion. Parents' everyday acts of microbiome care refused the divisions imposed by medical diagnoses and, instead, arced toward biosocial coalitions defined by and geared toward addressing harmful social experiences of disability and related structural determinants of health.

So far, it might seem like microbiome etiologies and associated practices of care arc toward a bright health future. However, there are risks when people and groups turn away from—or are pushed outside of—institutional medicine and take up unsanctioned, experimental health practices. By taking up microbiome care, Somali American participants entered a space of unregulated and uninsured alternative medicine. There was not a professional code of ethics or overseeing body to license and regulate their naturpathic providers and ensure that their care was safe and effective. There are certainly accounts of self-treating individuals and providers attempting microbiome therapies that are dangerous (Lorimer, 2017; Ekekezie et al., 2020). Microbiome care was expensive and was not reimbursable through insurance. In one interview, Nasra admitted, "Don't think I don't worry sometimes, is this all a scam? I'm spending money to put marijuana lotion on my child, to plan meals. It's a lot of money. But I'm the kind of person, I try everything. And it's been good" (10/12/2018). Five mothers turned toward unregulated, expensive, experimental therapies in large part because these liminal sorts of care could be practiced at home, with everyday materials, without institutional oversight and surveillance, and in response to parents' own stories, histories, and experiential insights, but there are grave risks that come with this freedom.

What to make of a rhetorical refusal that arcs toward collaborative, socially enmeshed, coalitional care but also to experimental, potentially exploitative, potentially harmful care? More simply, how to respond to medical dissent that is risky? To address this question, the next section advances a rhetorical framework, built from the previous five topoi, to listen to medical dissent, including dangerous and nonscientific medical dissent, as rhetorical refusal. The five topoi form a rhetorical framework useful to recognize rhetorical refusal and, in turn, reorient discussion from whether science is right or wrong to the murkier, more consequential, and highly uneven ways that science sediments into our everyday lives.

A Five-Topoi Framework for Listening to Medical Dissent as Rhetorical Refusal

Noncompliance, nonconcordance, nonadherence, hesitancy. Resistance, suspicion, refusal. These are the terms with which I opened this book, terms that scientists, healthcare providers, humanists, patients, and others have used to make sense of why some people do not follow medical recommendations and do not use available medical resources. I introduced rhetorical refusal into this set of frames and argued that rhetorical refusal offers something different largely because of its focus on and capacity for rhetoricity. Rhetorical refusal approaches dissent as communicative, agentive, and participatory. Rhetorical refusal listens for the deeper contexts that make dissent logical or preferable, listens to the unlikely futures that become sayable because of dissent. Rhetorical refusal surfaces dissent's exigences and the futures that dissent serves. But if we are to broaden the purview from whether the dissenter is right or wrong, if we are to look beyond the veracity of scientific facts and to instead consider how knowledge works in people's everyday lives and social worlds, then it's vital to have rhetorical infrastructure for these discussions. We need rhetorical tools to describe medical problems as, sometimes, social problems that call for social action (Hausman, 2019, p. 12). We need an "alternative vocabulary for framing the debate (as something other than science)" (Goldenberg, 2021, p. 107).

Indeed, Goldenberg (2021) has argued that our deliberative tools to discuss the social determinants and political dimensions of illness and health are diminished by an overvaluation of medical evidence, what Goldenberg terms an "evidence-based everything" discourse. There's an assumption that everything—policy, medicine, business, education, bioethics—should be grounded in evidence. If a decision is grounded in scientific evidence, it is correct and good action will follow (pp. 94–95). Goldenberg describes this apotheosis of evidence as "scientistic reductionism of socially complex issues like vaccine uptake and refusal" and calls for rhetorical interventions to unsettle the hallowed place of scientific evidence as a deliberative end-all-be-all (p. 98). Writes Goldenberg,

The legacies of science-based everything and scientized politics have made the language of science the currency of political discourse. Thus, opponents have little recourse for expressing disapproval other than challenging the science. To get past scientized politics and political stalemates, we need an alternative vocabulary for framing the debate (as something other than science) and venues for normative debate. (p. 107)

The five topoi described in this chapter build a framework to understand medical dissent outside "evidence-based everything" premises. They provide an "alternative vocabulary for framing the debate (as something other than science)."

Informed by Ratcliffe's theory of rhetorical listening (2005), this five-part framework is attuned to the logics that inform dissent instead of the specific claims that might constitute an act of dissent. This framework is useful for taking seriously the reasons, outside of scientific reasoning, that people subscribe to divergent, including nonscientific and not evidence-based, health epistemologies. Crucially, these topoi have little to do with science. They have nothing to do with whether a health claim is scientifically accurate or not. But they have much to do with how and why people apply or do not apply science in their lives. It was from these topoi—rather than arguments about science and evidence—that parents' distrust in medicine fermented and their microbiome beliefs flourished. As Hausman (2019) has shown and participating Somali American parents' stories have demonstrated, "what we do to our bodies in the service of health is never only an effect of data and scientific considerations" (p. 212). This five-part framework starts to map those other factors—not the data, evidence, and scientific considerations—that shape health decisions and beliefs.

The topoi identify five sites—medicine, care, affect, story, and social determinants of health—at which people grapple with science and medicine in their daily lives. In this study, different health epistemologies materialized in Somali American parents' lives at the levels of medicine (What medicines were available within this epistemology?), location (Where does care take place?), affect (How does healthcare feel? What are the relationships like?), story (Whose expertise matters? Where does lived experience and personal story fit in?), and social determinants of health (How does this epistemology acknowledge or not the interplay between body, history, environment, and power structures?). As a framework, these topoi center questions including the following: What are the medicines prescribed? How do people get them? How do they work with (or not) people's day-to-day lives? What space is there for collaboration? Where does care happen? What knowledges and subjectivities have epistemic power in this place? What does it feel like? Whose expertise is valued? What stories matter? What stories get bracketed? What does it mean for a child to thrive, for *my* child to thrive? What relationships become possible and impossible? Where is a health problem located, in an individual body, in social structures, or somewhere else? What power relationships are at play? What epistemologies "(finally) make space for us, its patients" or not? (Mol, 2008, p. 2).

At each of these sites, microbiome care descended into participating parents' everyday lives in ways that worked—in ways that meshed with parents' daily realities, affirmed parents' experiences, gave voice to parents' anxieties and hopes, and helped families thrive. These topoi direct discussion away from science and its facts and toward the "embedded questions" behind health decisions and beliefs, the questions that "are not amenable to what goes by the name of scientific reasoning" (Hausman, 2019, p. 214). Indeed, health decisions are not just logical decisions made from population-level evidence but are also "individual, embodied, material experiences," and so healthcare responses, even when grounded in evidence-based medicine, "demand deliberation, discussion, and understanding—all enactments of discourse that persuasion, and thus rhetoric, requires" (Lawrence, 2020, p. 3). The five topoi provide rhetorical infrastructure to listen to medical dissent outside of considerations of right and wrong beliefs. They provide a framework to listen to dissent as rhetorical refusal. And rhetorical refusal, as a concept, broadens the discussion to include not just the moment of dissent but its fertile ground and possible futures. These five topoi point to core sites that can either form the loam for rhetorical refusal or can flourish into strong relationships and communities where evidence-based medicine and scientific expertise make sense not just in the lab but in people's lived experiences. These five topoi provide a rhetorical infrastructure to listen to rhetorical refusal, to respond to the fertile ground of medical dissent, and to attune to the futures that dissent makes possible.

Conclusion

This book has followed the arc of participating Somali American parents' rhetorical refusals of the MMR vaccine to the microbiome. In the beginning of this chapter, I mapped mainstream scientific and public discourses of the microbiome. In these discourses, the microbiome reverberated with promise to radically reenvision the human body and its interdependence. But these discourses have been swiftly re-enfolded into traditional and harmful ways of conceiving of health as an individual responsibility and moral achievement; this neoliberal framing of health deepens structural inequities and systemic racism, often by disavowing race as a nonbiological category only to recuperate race as a biological explanatory factor for health disparities (Happe, 2013). Still, people who are marginalized by microbiome discourses also use microbiome discourses in inventive, restorative, and protective ways. In this chapter, Somali American participants took the framework of the embedded, ecosystem body and practiced care in which their lived experiences and histories were somaticized into actionable grounds for collective action. Mothers explained autism as the result of personal and collective histories: warfare, forced migration, home loss, refugee journeys—and ongoing precarity— structural racism, specific incidents of racism, sexism, Islamophobia, poverty, discrimination, access barriers, surveillance, and policing. The microbiome provided a scientific-adjacent discourse to identify autism as community sickness and outlined therapeutic practices to care for autism as such. Parents used microbiome discourses to locate past traumas in the body and to then attend to those traumas through caring for the body by means of diets, dirt, sunshine, migration, probiotics and prebiotics, and refusals of medical interventions. However, a key reason that participants found at-home care possible was that participants practiced a fringe microbiome medicine, one that operated outside of professional oversight or accountability. Somali American participants' uptake of the microbiome therefore also highlights the grave challenges that come with refusing medicine and vying for a different future.

But this tension—that the microbiome meshes with participants' lives, even as it might not be used to administer healthful interventions—is one reason why it is so important to attend to medical dissent as a rhetorical refusal. Doing so is one way to address the actual reasons that a person may turn away from medicine, with all its evidence and resources, and practice alternative forms of healthcare. The five topoi described in this chapter provide a portable rhetorical framework with which to listen to medical dissent, wrong explanations (for example, that the MMR vaccine can cause autism), mistakes, and non-uptake of medical tools and therapies as rhetorical refusals. These topoi broaden the purview from whether the dissenter is right or wrong; they provide instead a generative framework that follows how facts and knowledge descend into people's everyday lives and social worlds. The five topoi map sites that illuminate the experience of medicine, science, and knowledge in people's everyday lives. Beyond this study, this framework is useful to respond to other acts of dissent as a communicative, constrained, and insightful rhetorical refusals. Not as mistakes to be corrected but as openings for listening, collaboration, and change.

CONCLUSION

This study took shape amid a measles outbreak. Throughout the outbreak, one question seemed to be everywhere: Why were Somali American parents refusing the MMR vaccine? And it was followed by another question: How can public health departments get Somali American children vaccinated, and quickly? During my time working on this study, I heard many stories about Somali American parents, their medical noncompliance, and their unscientific health beliefs. Most accounts linked low MMR vaccination rates with unscientific fears about autism and its causation. In news media, in public health reports, and in conversations with healthcare providers, social service providers, and community health workers, I encountered frequent explanations for why Somali vaccination rates were low in Minnesota and why fears about autism persisted. Healthcare and social service professionals often proffered theories about Somali American parents' lack of education and consequential vulnerability to antivaccination appeals. I heard theories about Somali people's stubborn distrust of medicine and science and their misplaced faith in spiritual and holistic healing. I heard theories about cultural beliefs, mostly accounts of cultural taboo and stigma that attached to disability in Somali and East African cultures. I most often heard that there is not a word for autism in the Somali language. This anecdote was shorthand to explain that Somalis therefore did not know about autism and were prone to thinking that autism was unique to the US. In short, there were many explanations circulating about why Somali parents were declining vaccines. And in tandem with these explanations, there were many preset solutions, mostly health literacy outreach, mandated vaccination, and barrier removal.

These preset solutions all represent important goals, but I also wanted to ask: Why did dominant explanations for Somali American parents' MMR vaccine refusals focus so wholly on individual beliefs? What logics and histories inform dominant approaches to medical dissent as an irrational but remediable act of individual noncompliance? How has medical dissent been defined and explained elsewhere? And might there be significance to Somali Minnesotans' dissent? Might there be arguments, stories, histories, and ideas that were being written off because their external packaging was that of noncompliance? Because so many of us were locked into "evidence-based everything" thinking (Goldenberg, 2021)? Was there reason to listen to and follow this dissent, instead of—or in addition to—trying to quickly and permanently reverse it? What is the significance of Somali Minnesotan parents' expressions of dissent? These questions guided the writing of this book.

I began this book by considering the limited ways that medical dissent has been named and explained. Dissent, often approached on a gradient of noncompliance, is typically defined as a wrong but fixable stance. Sometimes there is room for understanding dissent as more than just illogical—for example, steep access barriers to medicine can erode trust, and cultural insensitivity can alienate patients. Always, though, compliance is the right answer, even if medical institutions and their leaders bear some of the responsibility for facilitating trusting, accessible spaces where compliance is logical and actionable (Goldenberg, 2021). This medical frame for approaching dissent works within and naturalizes a culture of biomedicine that "is often frustratingly inattentive to the weight history continues to bear on peoples of African descent as they counter and navigate neoliberal policies, mushrooming state-industry partnerships, and their pharmaceutical and technological offerings" (Charles, 2022, p. 171). Benjamin (2013) has referred to the biomedical framing of dissent as a persisting "inexplicable curiosity" as the work of "analytical summersaults" that biomedicine must undertake to avoid acknowledging that noncompliance is an obvious response to racism in medicine, an obvious response to a system wherein the benefits and risks are not evenly distributed (p. 140). Simply, dissent is logical. In response, Charles and Benjamin and fellow scholars have theorized dissent outside of a biomedical frame and set of premises (Lawrence, Hausman, and Dannenberg, 2014; Simpson, 2014; Sobo, 2015; Benjamin, 2016; Hausman, 2019; Lawrence, 2020; Charles, 2022; Goldenberg, 2021).

In line with this body of scholarship, Somali American parents' stories have given voice to a theory of rhetorical refusal. That is, to local, situated refusals that are participatory, protective, generative, and often defiantly hopeful. The rhetorical refusal is especially attuned to rhetorical strategies developed by marginalized persons who face day-to-day epistemic marginalization (Fricker, 2007; Yam, 2019). For these reasons, rhetorical refusals are not always readily recognizable as rhetorical acts. Throughout this book, I have identified rhetorical refusals that might otherwise be categorized as scientific errors, mistakes, moments of confusion, lapses in judgment, the unfortunate results of too-steep access barriers, or as simply nothing, a silence. These refusals are voiced in institutional, hierarchical spaces, wherein Somali parents have little access to voice, rhetorical platform, or ethos. These rhetorical refusals—a question left blank, a script left unfilled, a vaccine administered one year "late"—were everyday forms of interruption and disengagement that Somali American mothers used to protect their children within asymmetrical power relations, within medical systems informed by racist histories and exclusions, and in the face of uncertain health futures. The concept of rhetorical refusal marks these moments and then situates these rhetorical acts on an arc. In doing so, rhetorical refusal considers dissent as always informed by its contexts—by overlapping historical, sociopolitical, familial, embodied, and material contexts—and as striving for different futures.

I have used the rhetorical refusal to name acts of dissent as ethical, political, sometimes activist, sometimes affiliative, always protective moves. Chapter 1 followed why Somali American mothers continued to describe autism as community sickness, even after this group of mothers enrolled in and claimed to have learned and benefited from an autism-focused health literacy class. Community sickness was a rhetorical refusal enacted through alternative discourses. Participants developed alternative, nonstandard discourses of autism to insist on the ways that autism was a community sickness, a specific experience for Somali refugee families, one that could not and should not be subsumed in an abstracted, context-free medical account of autism. The slippages between autism and community sickness show, importantly, that rhetorical refusals do not always make activist and public-facing arguments, do not always strive for influence in spaces of public deliberation, do not always aim for policy change. Sometimes, rhetorical refusals turn inward. Sometimes, rhetorical refusals are useful to gather those who share a marginalized position and related experiences of precarity and illness (community sickness) and to support each other. In these instances, rhetorical refusal can serve an affiliative, in-group tactic geared toward care and protection. The discourse of community sickness, as a rhetorical refusal, was useful for Somali American parents to find each other and then find the language to discuss their lived experiences of autism and the adaptive tactics that helped them protect their children.

Moving into the formative measles outbreak, I argued that Somali American parents' vaccine hesitancy cannot be wholly explained by deficits in literacy, culture, and trust. The 2017 Minnesota measles outbreak was not a battle between public health professionals and antivaccination charlatans over the up-for-grabs beliefs of Somali American parents. Somali American parents' vaccine hesitations were informed by concerns specific to their experiences as refugees and racialized persons in the US. In turn, parents' refusals raised potentially legitimate health concerns—concerns about how seriously people, particularly those whose somatic experiences and backgrounds have not been included in medical research and whose needs have rarely been centered in medical care and public health policy, should take population-level medical evidence. Chapter 2 showed how rhetorical refusal can serve an important epistemic function: to identify potentially real health problems, contest scientific knowledge, and collaboratively advance medical knowledge.

In chapter 3, I approached Somali American mothers' so-called errors on the WCAG applications as rhetorical refusals. Somali American mothers refused to participate in bureaucratic procedures that assumed that all applicants related to the state as a neutral and beneficent actor. Somali mothers' refusals, for example, to describe a child on his worst day or to invite state assessors into their homes, insisted on accountability for the harmful ways that racialized mothers are surveilled, disciplined, policed, and judged as unfit mothers. As well, these refusals arced toward forms of care that were not supported by the WCAG, forms of care that did not regard autism as an individual impairment and that did not prioritize making a child measurably normal. Somali parents' written and rejected proposals envision what equitable, community-enmeshed care could look like. This chapter depicted how rhetorical refusals unfold in bureaucratic writing situations—where discourse is highly regulated and the stories applicants can tell very limited—and why, in these consequential spaces, listening for rhetorical refusals in silences, blank spaces, and mistakes is so crucial.

Lastly, the microbiome emerged as a discourse and set of practices that became possible after participants refused to wholly adopt the medical definitions of autism their health literacy teachers taught them, refused vaccines, and refused state-sponsored medical care. Five Somali mothers found in the microbiome a set of discourses, practices, and relationships through which they could care for autism as community sickness. Within microbiome-informed, naturopathic care, participants' personal and familial stories and experiences were key to diagnosis and treatment. Parents cared for their children not as children with autism, but as children of diaspora, children who had rich family histories ruptured by trauma, children with meaningful kin networks and genealogies, children with strengths and singular traits, and children whose care must attend to these specificities. The microbiome, as a scientific-adjacent discourse, was useful to parents to craft and occupy rhetorical subjectivities with which they could make arguments about community sickness and about what care for community sickness looked like. This kind of care involved biosocial communities and collective action more so than individual therapeutics. Across participants' stories about the microbiome and their heterogenous autism etiologies emerged five topoi. These topoi map the sites at which discourses of health and medicine descended into participants' daily lives and social worlds, and they provide rhetorical infrastructure to discuss health decisions and beliefs outside of whether there is science to back them. At the end of this chapter, I advanced this five-part framework as a portable, rhetorical tool useful to listen to medical dissent and noncompliance as rhetorical refusal. Rhetorical refusal turns the discussion away from how to convert noncompliance into compliance and toward the harder but essential questions about the fertile ground that continues to sustain dissent and the futures that are more important to some dissenters than the immediate benefits of medicine.

Together, these chapters voice a call, ultimately, to listen. This book is a study of one specific, nongeneralizable series of refusals that occurred in the wake of a measles outbreak and in a specific sociopolitical context and within specific families. This specificity is not a detriment but is key to listening to and learning from rhetorical refusals (Lawrence, Hausman, and Dannenberg, 2014). This book is a call for granular, qualitative, ethnographic research approaches that listen to participants as inherently informed and knowledgeable. Listening to rhetorical refusals—as well as ethnographic refusals (Simpson, 2014), affiliative refusal (Sobo, 2016), biodefection (Benjamin, 2016), suspicion (Charles, 2022)—involves sustained engagement with local communities and their health beliefs, even when these beliefs are informed by nonscientific epistemologies. Listening involves following acts of dissent as rhetorical refusals that can envision radically different ways of practicing care and facilitating community health. This book offers the concept of rhetorical refusal and a call to continue to listen to the cultural logics that inform health claims (Ratcliffe, 2005). Across these four sites covered in each of this book's four chapters, rhetorical refusal surfaces care's inequalities and the political and ethical stakes of public health and medical practices. Rhetorical refusal, mapped along an arc, reveals the broader terrain of medical dissent. Rhetorical refusal reveals how not just scientific fact but also healthcare infrastructure, biomedical authority, social services, documentation, state priorities and processes, family history and lore, and histories of medical injustice all have a role to play in health beliefs and decisions. Each refusal occurs on its own irreducible arc. But continuing to voice, listen to, learn from, and follow refusals can build theory that accounts for multiple epistemologies of health and illness and, especially, the adaptive practices of those whose needs, embodiments, and histories have not been centered, cared for, or trusted in mainstream medical discourses. Listening to rhetorical refusals and following their arcs can continue to build a participatory, polyvocal map of health, science, illness, and care and can, in turn, build healthy communities.

REFERENCES

Abdi, C. M. (2014). Threatened identities and gendered opportunities: Somali migration to America. *Signs: Journal of Women in Culture and Society, 39*(2), 459–483. https://doi.org/10.1086/673380

Abdi, C. M. (2015a). Disclaimed or reclaimed? Muslim refugee youth and belonging in the age of hyperbolisation. *Journal of Intercultural Studies, 36*(5), 564–578. https://doi.org/10.1080/07256868.2015.1072905

Abdi, C. M. (2015b). *Elusive Jannah: The Somali diaspora and a borderless Muslim identity*. University of Minnesota Press.

Agboka, G. Y. (2013). Participatory localization: A social justice approach to navigating unenfranchised/disenfranchised cultural sites. *Technical Communication Quarterly, 22*(1), 28–49. https://doi.org/10.1080/10572252.2013.730966

AHRQ (2008). America's health literacy: Why we need accessible health information. https://www.ahrq.gov/sites/default/files/wysiwyg/health-literacy/dhhs-2008-issue-brief.pdf

Alaimo, S. (2010). *Bodily natures: Science, environment, and the material self*. Indiana University Press.

Allen-Vercoe E. (2013). Bringing the gut microbiota into focus through microbial culture: recent progress and future perspective. *Current opinion in microbiology, 16*(5), 625–629. https://doi.org/10.1016/j.mib.2013.09.008

American Hospital Association. (2016). Hospitals caring for their communities. https://www.aha.org/news/headline/2016-02-18-hospitals-caring-their-communities

Anand, R., & Winters, M. (2008). A retrospective view of corporate diversity training from 1964 to the present. *Academy of Management Learning & Education, 7*(3), 356–372.

Aronson, J. K. (2007). Compliance, concordance, adherence. *British Journal of Clinical Pharmacology, 63*(4), 383–384. https://doi.org/10.1111/j.1365-2125.2007.02893.x

Autism Self Advocacy Network. (2022). ASAN Comments on Section 1557. https://autisticadvocacy.org/2022/10/asan-comments-on-section-1557/

Banerjee, E., Griffith, J., Kenyon, C., Christianson, B., Strain, A., Martin, K., McMahon, M., Bagstad, E., Laine, E., Hardy, K., Grilli, G., Walters, J., Dunn, D., Roddy, M., & Ehresmann, K. (2020). Containing a measles outbreak in Minnesota, 2017: Methods and challenges. *Perspectives in Public Health, 140*(3), 162–171. https://doi.org/10.1177/1757913919871072

Belluz, J. (2017). Minnesota is fighting its largest measles outbreak in nearly 30 years. Blame vaccine deniers. *Vox.* https://www.vox.com/2017/5/8/15577316/minnesota-measles-outbreak-explained

Bellware, K. (2017). Doctors weren't listening to Somali immigrants' autism concerns. Then antivaxxers did. *Huffington Post.* https://www.huffingtonpost.com/entry/minnesota-measles-outbreak_us_591224dfe4b05e1ca202a154

Benezra, A. (2020). Race in the microbiome. *Science, Technology, & Human Values, 45*(5), 877–902. https://doi.org/10.1177/0162243920911998

Benezra, A. (2021). Microbial kin: Relations of environment and time. *Medical Anthropology Quarterly, 35*(4), 511–528. https://doi.org/10.1111/maq.12680

Benjamin, R. (2013). *People's science: Bodies and rights on the stem cell frontier.* Stanford University Press.

Benjamin, R. (2016). Informed refusal: Toward a justice-based bioethics. *Science, Technology, & Human Values, 41*(6), 967–990.

Berns-McGown, R. (1999). *Muslims in the diaspora.* University of Toronto Press.

Betancourt, J. R., Green, A. R., Carrillo, J. E., & Ananeh-Firempong, O. (2003). Defining cultural competence: A practical framework for addressing racial/ethnic disparities in health and health care. *Public Health Reports, 118*(4), 293–302. https://doi.org/10.1016/s0033-3549(04)50253-4

Betancourt, J. R., Green, A. R., Carrillo, J. E., & Park, E. R. (2005). Cultural competence and health care disparities: Key perspectives and trends. *Health Affairs, 24*(2), 499–510. https://doi.org/10.1377/hlthaff.24.2.499

Bichell, R. E. (2015). Clinical trials still don't reflect the diversity of America. *NPR.* https://www.npr.org/sections/health-shots/2015/12/16/459666750/clinical-trials-still-dont-reflect-the-diversity-of-america

Blaser, M. (2011). Stop the killing of beneficial bacteria. *Nature, 476,* 393–394. https://doi.org/10.1038/476393a

Blaser, M. (2014). *Missing microbes: How the overuse of antibiotics is fueling our modern plagues.* Henry Holt.

Bloom-Pojar, R. (2018). *Translanguaging outside the Academy: Negotiating rhetoric and healthcare in the Spanish Caribbean.* Conference on College Composition and Communication / National Council of Teachers of English.

Branswell, H. (2017). Measles sweeps an immigrant community targeted by antivaccine activists. https://www.statnews.com/2017/05/08/measles-vaccines-somali/

Britt, E. (2018). *Reimagining advocacy: Rhetorical education in the legal clinic.* Pennsylvania State University Press.

Brody, J. (2017). Unlocking the secretes of the microbiome. *New York Times.* https://www.nytimes.com/2017/11/06/well/live/unlocking-the-secrets-of-the-microbiome.html

Brown, P. (2007). *Toxic exposures: Contested illnesses and the environmental health movement.* Columbia University Press.

Brown, P., Mayer, B., Zavestoski, S., Luebke, T., Mandelbaum, J., & McCormick, S. (2004). Clearing the air and breathing freely: The health politics of air pollution and asthma. *International Journal of Health Services, 34*(1), 39–63. https://doi.org/10.2190/D7QX-Q3FQ-BJUG-EVHL

Brown, P., & Mikkelsen, E. J. (1998). *No safe place: Toxic waste, leukemia, and community action.* University of California Press.

Campeau, K. (2019). Vaccine barriers, vaccine refusals: Situated vaccine decision-making in the wake of the 2017 Minnesota measles outbreak. *Rhetoric of Health & Medicine, 2*(2), 176–207. https://doi.org/10.5744/rhm.2019.1007

Canto, J. G., Goldberg, R. J., Hand, M. M., Bonow, R. O., Sopko, G., Pepine, C. J., & Long, T. (2007). Symptom presentation of women with acute coronary syndromes: Myth vs reality. *Archives of Internal Medicine, 167*(22), 2405–2413. https://doi.org/10.1001/archinte.167.22.2405

Centers for Disease Control and Prevention (CDC). (2020). Narcolepsy following 2009 Pandemrix influenza vaccination in Europe. https://www.cdc.gov/vaccinesafety/concerns/history/narcolepsy-flu.html

Chamberlain, S. (2017). Minnesota measles outbreak: Officials say Somali families 'targeted with misinformation.' Fox News. https://www.foxnews.com/health/minnesota-measles-outbreak-officials-say-somali-families-targeted-with-misinformation

Charles, N. (2018). HPV vaccination and affective suspicions in Barbados. *Feminist Formations, 30*(1), 46–70. https://doi.org/10.1353/ff.2018.0003

Charles, N. (2022). *Suspicion: Vaccines, hesitancy, and the affective politics of protection in Barbados.* Duke University Press.

Clare, E. (2017). *Brilliant imperfections: Grappling with cure.* Duke University Press.

Clayton, J., & Collins, F. S. (2014). Policy: NIH to balance sex in cell and animal studies. *Nature, 509,* 282–283. https://doi.org/10.1038/509282a

Cohen, J. J., Gabriel, B. A., & Terrell, C. (2002). The case for diversity in the health care workforce. *Health Affairs, 21*(5), 90–102. https://doi.org/10.1377/hlthaff.21.5.90

Collins, H. M., & Evans, R. (2002). The third wave of science studies: Studies of expertise and experience. *Social Studies of Science, 32*(2), 235–296. https://doi.org/10.1177/0306312702032002003

Collins, P. H. (1990). *Black feminist thought: Knowledge consciousness, and the politics of empowerment.* Routledge.

Conis, E. (2014). *Vaccine nation: America's changing relationship with immunizations.* University of Chicago Press.

Conis, E., & Hoenicke, S. (2022). Measles, media and memory: Journalism's role in framing collective memory of disease. *Journal of Medical Humanities, 43*(3), 405–420. https://doi.org/10.1007/s10912-021-09705-2

Conrad, P. (1985). The meaning of medications: Another look at compliance. *Social Science and Medicine, 20*(1), 29–37. https://doi.org/10.1016/0277-9536(85)90308-9

Cooper-Patrick, L., Gallo, J. J., Gonzales, J. J., Vu, H. T., Powe, N. R., Nelson, C., & Ford, D. E. (1999). Race, gender, and partnership in the patient-physician relationship. *JAMA, 282*(6), 583–589. https://doi.org/10.1001/jama.282.6.583

Cox, M. B. (2019). Working closets: Mapping queer professional discourses and why professional communication studies need queer rhetorics. *Journal of Business and Technical Communication, 33*(1), 1–25. https://doi.org/10.1177/105065191879869

Dasgupta, S. (2015). Medicalization. In R. Adams, B. Reiss, & D. Serlin (Eds.), *Keywords in disability studies* (pp. 120–121). New York University Press.

Davis, L. J. (1995). *Enforcing normalcy: Disability, deafness, and the body.* Verso.

Davis, M. S. (1968). Physiologic, psychological and demographic factors in patient compliance with doctors' orders. *Medical Care, 6*(2), 115–122. https://doi.org/10.1097/00005650-196803000-00003

Decoteau, C. L. (2017). The "Western disease": Autism and Somali parents' embodied health movements. *Social Science & Medicine (1982), 177,* 169–176. https://doi.org/10.1016/j.socscimed.2017.01.064

Decoteau, C. L. (2021). *The Western disease: Contesting autism in the Somali diaspora.* University of Chicago Press.

Derkatch, C. (2016). *Bounding biomedicine: Evidence and rhetoric in the new science of alternative medicine.* University of Chicago Press.

Derkatch, C. (2022). *Why wellness sells: Natural health in a pharmaceutical culture.* Johns Hopkins University Press.

Dolmage, J. T. (2014). *Disability Rhetoric.* Syracuse University Press.

Dorpenyo, I. K. (2022). Local knowledge as illiterate rhetoric: An antenarrative approach to enacting socially just technical communication. *Journal of Technical Writing and Communication, 52*(3), 291–315. https://doi.org/10.1177/00472816211030199

Downing, R., & Kowal, E. (2011). A postcolonial analysis of indigenous cultural awareness training for health workers. *Health Sociology Review, 20*(1), 5–15. https://doi.org/10.5172/hesr.2011.20.1.5

Dumes, A. A. (2020). *Divided bodies: Lyme disease, contested illness, and evidence-based medicine.* Duke University Press.

Duster T. (2006). The molecular reinscription of race: Unanticipated issues in biotechnology and forensic science. *Patterns of Prejudice, 40*(4–5), 427–441. https://doi.org/10.1080/00313220601020148

Dyer, O. (2017). Measles outbreak in Somali American community follows anti-vaccine talks. *BMJ, 357,* j2378–j2378. https://doi.org/10.1136/bmj.j2378

Edenfield, A. C., Holmes, S., & Colton, J. S. (2019). Queering tactical technical communication: DIY HRT. *Technical Communication Quarterly, 28*(3), 177–191. https://doi.org/10.1080/10572252.2019.1607906

Ekekezie, C., Perler, B. K., Wexler, A., Duff, C., Lillis, C. J., & Kelly, C. R. (2020). Understanding the scope of do-it-yourself fecal microbiota transplant. *American Journal of Gastroenterology, 115*(4), 603–607. https://doi.org/10.14309/ajg.0000000000000499

Epstein, S. (1996). *Impure science: AIDS, activism, and the politics of knowledge.* University of California Press.

Epstein, S. (2007). *Inclusion: The politics of difference in medical research.* University of Chicago Press.

Eyal, G., Hart, B., Onculer, E., Oren, N., & Rossi, N. (2010). *The autism matrix: The social origins of the autism epidemic.* Polity Press.

Fejerman, L., Ahmadiyeh, N., Hu, D., Huntsman, S., Beckman, K. B., Caswell, J. L., Tsung, K., John, E. M., Torres-Mejia, G., Carvajal-Carmona, L., Echeverry, M. M., Tuazon, A. M., Ramirez, C., Gignoux, C. R., Eng, C., Gonzalez-Burchard, E., Henderson, B., Le Marchand, L., Kooperberg, C., . . . Ziv, E. (2014). Genome-wide association study of breast cancer in Latinas identifies novel protective variants on 6q25. *Nature Communications, 5,* Article 5260. https://doi.org/10.1038/ncomms6260

Fettweis, J. M., Serrano, M. G., Brooks, J. P., Edwards, D. J., Girerd, P. H., Parikh, H. I., Huang, B., Arodz, T. J., Edupuganti, L., Glascock, A. L., Xu, J., Jimenez, N. R., Vivadelli, S. C., Fong, S. S., Sheth, N. U., Jean, S., Lee, V., Bokhari, Y. A., Lara, A. M., . . . Buck, G. A. (2019). The vaginal microbiome and preterm birth. *Nature Medicine, 25*(6), 1012–1021. https://doi.org/10.1038/s41591-019-0450-2

Finlay, B. B., & Arrieta, M. C. (2016). *Let them eat dirt: Saving your child from an oversanitized world*. Algonquin Books.

Fisher, J. A. (2020). *Adverse events: Race, inequality, and the testing of new pharmaceuticals*. New York University Press.

Fricker, M. (2007). *Epistemic injustice: Power and the ethics of knowing*. Oxford University Press.

Garrison-Joyner, V., & Caravella, E. (2020). Lapses in literacy: Cultural accessibility in graphic health communication. *Technical Communication Quarterly, 29*(3), iii–xxv. https://doi.org/10.1080/10572252.2020.1768295

Gehrig, J. L., Venkatesh, S., Chang, H. W., Hibberd, M. C., Kung, V. L., Cheng, J., Chen, R. Y., Subramanian, S., Cowardin, C. A., Meier, M. F., O'Donnell, D., Talcott, M., Spears, L. D., Semenkovich, C. F., Henrissat, B., Giannone, R. J., Hettich, R. L., Ilkayeva, O., Muehlbauer, M., Newgard, C. B., . . . Gordon, J. I. (2019). Effects of microbiota-directed foods in gnotobiotic animals and undernourished children. *Science, 365*(6449), eaau4732. https://doi.org/10.1126/science.aau4732

Gele, A. A., Pettersen, K. S., Torheim, L. E., & Kumar, B. (2016). Health literacy: The missing link in improving the health of Somali immigrant women in Oslo. *BMC Public Health, 16*(1), 1134. https://doi.org/10.1186/s12889-016-3790-6

Giddens, A. (1990). *The consequences of modernity*. Polity.

Gilbert, J. A., Blaser, M. J., Caporaso, J. G., Jansson, J. K., Lynch, S. V., & Knight, R. (2018). Current understanding of the human microbiome. *Nature Medicine, 24*(4), 392–400. https://doi.org/10.1038/nm.4517

Gilbert, J. A., Knight, R., & Blakeslee, S. (2017). *Dirt is good: The advantage of germs for your child's developing immune system*. Macmillan.

Glabau, D. (2022). *Food allergy advocacy: Parenting and the politics of care*. New York University Press.

Glenn, C. (2004). *Unspoken: A rhetoric of silence*. Southern Illinois University Press.

Goldenberg, M. (2021). *Vaccine hesitancy: Public trust, expertise, and the war on science*. University of Pittsburgh Press.

Gouge, C. (2018). "'The inconvenience of meeting you': Rereading non/compliance, enabling care." In A. K. Booher & J. Jung (Eds.), *Feminist rhetorical science studies* (pp. 114–140). Southern Illinois University Press.

Green, M. (2021). Resistance as participation: Queer theory's applications for HIV health technology design. *Technical Communication Quarterly, 30*(4), 331–344. https://doi.org/10.1080/10572252.2020.1831615

Greene, J. A. (2004). Therapeutic infidelities: 'Noncompliance' enters the medical literature, 1955–1975. *Social History of Medicine, 17*(3), 327–343. https://doi.org/10.1093/shm/17.3.327

Greenwood, B. N., Hardeman, R. R., Huang, L., & Sojourner, A. (2020). Physician–patient racial concordance and disparities in birthing mortality for newborns. *Proceedings of the National Academy of Sciences—PNAS, 117*(35), 21194–21200. https://doi.org/10.1073/pnas.1913405117

Hall, V., Banerjee, E., Kenyon, C., Strain, A., Griffith, J., Como-Sabetti, K., Heath, J., Bahta, L., Martin, K., McMahon, M., Johnson, D., Roddy, M., Dunn, D., & Ehresmann, K. (2017). Measles outbreak—Minnesota April–May 2017. *MMWR: Morbidity and Mortality Weekly Report, 66*(27), 713–717. https://doi.org/10.15585/mmwr.mm6627a1

Hallberg, P., Smedje, H., Eriksson, N., Kohnke, H., Daniilidou, M., Öhman, I., Yue, Q. Y., Cavalli, M., Wadelius, C., Magnusson, P. K. E., Landtblom, A. M., & Wadelius, M. (2019).

Pandemrix-induced narcolepsy is associated with genes related to immunity and neuronal survival. *EBioMedicine, 40,* 595–604. https://doi.org/10.1016/j.ebiom.2019.01.041

Hammitt, L. (2019). Haemophilus influenzae type b in Native American children. Centers for Disease Control and Prevention. ACIP Meeting Combination Vaccine, 201901(010503). https://stacks.cdc.gov/view/cdc/7808

Hamraie, A. (2017). *Building access: Universal design and the politics of disability.* University of Minnesota Press.

Happe, K. (2013). *The material gene: Gender, race, and heredity after the Human Genome Project.* New York University Press.

Harper, K. C. (2021). Tired as a mutha: Black mother activists and the fight for affordable housing and health care. *Technical Communication Quarterly, 30*(3), 230–240. https://doi.org/10.1080/10572252.2021.1930183

Hartman, S. V. (2007). *Lose your mother: A journey along the Atlantic slave route.* Farrar, Strauss, and Giroux.

Hausman, B. L. (2017). Immunity, modernity, and the biopolitics of vaccination. *Configurations, 25*(3), 279–300. https://dx.doi.org/10.1353/con.2017.0020

Hausman, B. L. (2019). *Anti/vax: Reframing the vaccination controversy.* Cornell University Press.

Hausman, B. L. (2022). Hausman on Goldenberg, 'Vaccine Hesitancy: Public Trust, Expertise, and the War on Science.' *H-Net Network on Science, Medicine, and Technology.* https://networks.h-net.org/node/9782/reviews/10246600/hausman-goldenberg-vaccine-hesitancy-public-trust-expertise-and-war

Hausman, B. L., Lawrence, H. Y., Marmagas, S. W., Fortenberry, L., & Dannenberg, C. J. (2020). H1N1 vaccination and health beliefs in a rural community in the southeastern United States: Lessons learned. *Critical Public Health, 30*(2), 245–251. https://doi.org/10.1080/09581596.2018.1546825

Hayden, C. (2003). *When nature goes public: The making and unmaking of bioprospecting in Mexico.* Princeton University Press.

Heier, M. S., Gautvik, K. M., Wannag, E., Bronder, K. H., Midtlyng, E., Kamaleri, Y., & Storsaeter, J. (2013). Incidence of narcolepsy in Norwegian children and adolescents after vaccination against H1N1 influenza A. *Sleep Medicine, 14*(9), 867–871. https://doi.org/10.1016/j.sleep.2013.03.020

Herring, S., Spangaro, J., Lauw, M., & McNamara, L. (2013). The intersection of trauma, racism, and cultural competence in effective work with aboriginal people: Waiting for trust. *Australian Social Work, 66*(1), 104–117. https://doi.org/10.1080/0312407X.2012.697566

Hewitt, A., Gulaid, A., Hamre, K., Esler, P., Reichle, J., & Reiff, M. (2013). Minneapolis Somali autism spectrum disorder prevalence project. University of Minnesota Institute on Community Integration. https://ici.umn.edu/products/583

Hewitt, A., Hall-Lande, J., Hamre, K., Esler, A. N., Punyko, J., Reichle, J., & Gulaid, A. A. (2016). Autism spectrum disorder (ASD) prevalence in Somali and non-Somali children. *Journal of Autism and Developmental Disorders, 46*(8), 2599–2608. https://doi.org/10.1007/s10803-016-2793-6

Hickey, K. T., Masterson Creber, R. M., Reading, M., Sciacca, R. R., Riga, T. C., Frulla, A. P., & Casida, J. M. (2018). Low health literacy: Implications for managing cardiac patients in practice. *The Nurse Practitioner, 43*(8), 49–55. https://doi.org/10.1097/01.NPR.0000541468.54290.49

Hobson-West, P. (2007). 'Trusting blindly can be the biggest risk of all': Organised resistance to childhood vaccination in the UK. *Sociology of Health & Illness, 29*(2), 198–215. https://doi.org/10.1111/j.1467-9566.2007.00544.x

Hochschild, A. R. (2020). *Strangers in their own land.* New Press.

Hoffmann, D. E., & Tarzian, A. J. (2001). The girl who cried pain: A bias against women in the treatment of pain. *Journal of Law, Medicine & Ethics, 28*(s4), 13–27. https://doi.org/10.1111/j.1748-720X.2001.tb00037.x

Holladay, D. (2017). Classified conversations: Psychiatry and tactical technical communication in online spaces. *Technical Communication Quarterly, 26*(1), 8–24. https://doi.org/10.1080/10572252.2016.1257744

Horst, C. M. A. (2006). Buufis amongst Somalis in Dadaab: The transnational and historical logics behind resettlement dreams. *Journal of Refugee Studies, 19*(2), 143–157. https://doi.org/10.1093/jrs/fej017

Howard, J. (2017). Antivaccine groups blamed in Minnesota measles outbreak. *CNN.* https://www.cnn.com/2017/05/08/health/measles-minnesota-somali-anti-vaccine-bn/index.html

Howatt, G., & Mahamud, F. (2017). Antivaccine groups step up outreach to Minnesota Somali families over measles outbreak. *Star Tribune.* http://www.startribune.com/in-minnesota-measles-outbreak-health-officials-fight-a-two-front-war/420786463/

Ireson, J., Taylor, A., Richardson, E., Greenfield, B., & Jones, G. (2022). Exploring invisibility and epistemic injustice in long COVID—A citizen science qualitative analysis of patient stories from an online COVID community. *Health Expectations: An International Journal of Public Participation in Health Care and Health Policy, 25*(4), 1753–1765. https://doi.org/10.1111/hex.13518

Jack, J. (2014). *Autism and gender: From refrigerator mothers to computer geeks.* University of Illinois Press.

Johnson, J., & Kennedy, K. (2020). Introduction: Disability, in/visibility, and risk. *Rhetoric Society Quarterly, 50*(3), 161–165. https://doi.org/10.1080/02773945.2020.1752126

Jones, N. N., Moore, K. R., & Walton, R. (2016). Disrupting the Past to Disrupt the Future: An Antenarrative of Technical Communication. *Technical Communication Quarterly, 25*(4), 211–229. https://doi.org/10.1080/10572252.2016.1224655

Jongen, C., McCalman, J., & Bainbridge, R. (2018). Health workforce cultural competency interventions: A systematic scoping review. *BMC Health Services Research, 18*(1), 232. https://doi.org/10.1186/s12913-018-3001-5

Kafer, A. (2013). *Feminist, queer, crip.* Indiana University Press.

Kang, D., Adams, J. B., Gregory, A. C., Borody, T., Chittick, L., Fasano, A., Khoruts, A., Geis, E., Maldonado, J., McDonough-Means, S., Pollard, E. L., Roux, S., Sadowsky, M. J., Lipson, K. S., Sullivan, M. B., Caporaso, J. G., & Krajmalnik-Brown, R. (2017). Microbiota transfer therapy alters gut ecosystem and improves gastrointestinal and autism symptoms: An open-label study. *Microbiome, 5*(1). https://doi.org/10.1186/s40168-016-0225-7.

Keene Woods N., Ali, U., Medina, M., Reyes, J., Chesser, A. K. (2023). Health literacy, health outcomes and equity: A trend analysis based on a population survey. *Journal of Primary Care & Community Health, 14* (21501319231156132). https://doi.org/10.1177/21501319231156132

Keränen, L. (2007). "Cause someday we all die": Rhetoric, agency, and the case of the "patient" preferences worksheet. *Quarterly Journal of Speech, 93*(2), 179–210.

Kerschbaum, S. L. (2014). On rhetorical agency and disclosing disability in academic writing. *Rhetoric Review, 33*(1), 55–71. https://doi.org/10.1080/07350198.2014.856730

Khazan, O. (2014). Wealthy white schools' vaccination rates are as low as South Sudan's. *The Atlantic.* https://www.theatlantic.com/health/archive/2014/09/wealthy-la-schools-vaccination-rates-are-as-low-as-south-sudans/380252/

Kickbusch, I., Pelikan, J. M, Apfel, F., & Tsouros, A. D. (2013). *Health literacy: The solid facts.* World Health Organization. https://apps.who.int/iris/handle/10665/326432

Kim, E. (2017). *Curative violence: Rehabilitating disability, gender, and sexuality in modern Korea.* Duke University Press.

Kimura, A. H. (2016). *Radiation brain moms and citizen scientists: The gender politics of food contamination after Fukushima.* Duke University Press.

Kleist, N., & Thorsen, D. (2016). *Hope and uncertainty in contemporary African migration.* Routledge.

Kline, W. (2010). *Bodies of knowledge: Sexuality, reproduction, and women's health in the Second Wave.* University of Chicago Press.

Kluchin, R. (2009). *Fit to be tied: Sterilization and reproductive right, 1950–1980.* Rutgers University Press.

Koerber, A. (2013). *Breast or bottle: Contemporary controversies in infant-feeding policy and practice.* University of South Carolina Press.

Kolodziejski, L. R. (2020). Beyond the "hullabaloo" of the vaccine "debate": Understanding parents' assessment of risks when making vaccine decisions. *Rhetoric of Health & Medicine,* 3(1), 63–92. https://doi.org/10.5744/rhm.2020.1003

Konrad, A. (2018). Reimagining work: Normative commonplaces and their effects on accessibility in workplaces. *Business and Professional Communication Quarterly,* 81(1), 123–141. https://doi.org/10.1177/2329490617752577

Kumar, S. B., Arnipalli, S. R., & Ziouzenkova, O. (2020). Antibiotics in food chain: The consequences for antibiotic resistance. *Antibiotics,* 9(10), 688. https://doi.org/10.3390/antibiotics9100688

Larson, H. (2020). *Stuck: How vaccine rumors start—and why they don't go away.* Oxford University Press.

Lawrence, H. Y. (2020). *Vaccine Rhetorics.* The Ohio State University Press.

Lawrence, H. Y., Hausman, B. L., & Dannenberg, C. J. (2014). Reframing medicine's publics: The local as a public of vaccine refusal. *Journal of Medical Humanities,* 35(2), 111–129. https://doi.org/10.1007/s10912-014-9278-4

Lay, M. (2000). *The rhetoric of midwifery: Gender, knowledge, and power.* Rutgers University Press.

Leach, M., & Fairhead, J. (2008). *Vaccine anxieties: Global science, child health, and society.* Routledge.

Leavitt, J. W. (1986). *Brought to bed: Childbearing in America, 1750 to 1950.* Oxford University Press.

Leeds, M., & Muscoplat, M. (2017). Timeliness of receipt of early childhood vaccinations among children of immigrants—Minnesota, 2016. *Morbidity and Mortality Weekly Report,* 66(42), 1125–1129.

Lekas, H. M., Pahl, K., & Fuller Lewis, C. (2020). Rethinking cultural competence: Shifting to cultural humility. *Health services insights,* 13. https://doi.org/10.1177/1178632920970580

Li, J., Zhao, F., Wang, Y., Chen, J., Tao, J., Tian, G., Wu, S., Liu, W., Cui, Q., Geng, B., Zhang, W., Weldon, R., Auguste, K., Yang, L., Liu, X., Chen, L., Yang, X., Zhu, B., & Cai, J. (2017). Gut microbiota dysbiosis contributes to the development of hypertension. *Microbiome,* 5(1), 14. https://doi.org/10.1186/s40168-016-0222-x

Linton, S. (1998). *Claiming disability: Knowledge and identity.* New York University Press.

Livingston, J. (2005). *Debility and the moral imagination in Botswana.* Indiana University Press.

Lorimer, J. (2017). Probiotic environmentalities: Rewilding with wolves and worms. *Theory, Culture & Society,* 34(4), 27–48. https://doi.org/10.1177/0263276417695866

Lorimer, J. (2019). Hookworms make us human: The microbiome, eco-immunology, and a probiotic turn in Western health care. *Medical Anthropology Quarterly, 33*(1), 60–79. https://doi.org/10.1111/maq.12466

Luhmann, N. (1979). *Trust and power: Two works by Niklas Luhmann*. John Wiley.

Luzupone, C., Stombaugh, J., Gordon, J. I., Jansson, J. K., & Knight, R. (2012). Diversity, stability and resilience of the human gut microbiota. *Nature, 489*, 220–230. https://doi.org/10.1038/nature11550

MacFabe, D. F. (2013). Autism: Metabolism, mitochondria, and the microbiome. *Global Advances in Health and Medicine, 2*(6), 52–66. https://doi.org/10.7453/gahmj.2013.089

MacFabe, D. F. (2015). Enteric short-chain fatty acids: Microbial messengers of metabolism, mitochondria, and mind: Implications in autism spectrum disorders. *Microbial Ecology in Health and Disease, 26*(1), 28177–28177. https://doi.org/10.3402/mehd.v26.28177

Maenner, M. J., et al. (2021). Prevalence and Characteristics of Autism Spectrum Disorder Among Children Aged 8 Years—Autism and Developmental Disabilities Monitoring Network, 11 Sites, United States, 2018. *Morbidity and Mortality Weekly Report. Surveillance Summaries, 70*(11), 1–16. https://doi.org/10.15585/mmwr.ss7011a1

Mansh, M., Garcia, G., & Lunn, M. R. (2015). From patients to providers: Changing the culture in medicine toward sexual and gender minorities. *Academic Medicine, 90*(5), 574–580. https://doi.org/10.1097/ACM.0000000000000656

Marchesi, J. R., & Ravel, J. (2015). The vocabulary of microbiome research: A proposal. *Microbiome, 3*(1), 31–33. https://doi.org/10.1186/s40168-015-0094-5

Martin, E. (1994). *Flexible bodies: The role of immunity in American culture from the days of polio to the age of AIDS*. Routledge.

Martinez, A. Y. (2014). A plea for critical race theory counterstory: Stock story versus counterstory dialogues concerning Alejandra's "fit" in the academy. *Composition Studies, 42*(2), 33–47.

Martinez, A. Y. (2020). *Counterstory: The rhetoric and writing of critical race theory*. NCTE.

Martins, D. S. (2006). Compliance rhetoric and the impoverishment of context. *Communication Theory, 15*(1), 59–77. https://doi.org/10.1111/j.1468-2885.2005.tb00326.x

McCormick, S., Brody, J., Brown, P., & Polk, R. (2004). Public involvement in breast cancer research: An analysis and model for future research. *International Journal of Health Services, 34*(4), 625–646. https://doi.org/10.2190/HPXB-9RK8-ETVM-RVEA

McGranahan, C. (2016). Theorizing refusal: An introduction. *Cultural Anthropology, 31*(3), 319–325. https://doi.org/10.14506/ca31.3.01

McRuer, R. (2010). Compulsory able-bodiedness and queer/disabled existence. In L. J. Davis (Ed.), *The disability studies reader* (pp. 383–392). Routledge.

Meyer, P. A., Yoon, P. W., & Kaufmann, R. B. (2013). CDC health disparities and inequalities report—United States, 2013. *MMWR supplements, 62*(3), 3–5.

Minnesota Department of Health (MDH). (2009). Autism spectrum disorders among preschool children participating in Minneapolis Public Schools Early Childhood Special Education Programs. http://www.leg.state.mn.us/docs/2009/other/090520.pdf

Minnesota Health Literacy Partnership (2016). Bridging the gap: Taking action on health literacy in Minnesota. https://mn.gov/mnsure-stat/assets/2016-03-24-Health-Literacy-Presentation.pdf

Mipatrini, D., Stefanelli, P., Severoni, S., & Rezza, G. (2017). Vaccinations in migrants and refugees: A challenge for European health systems; A systematic review of current scientific evidence. *Pathogens and Global Health, 111*(2), 59–68. https://doi.org/10.1080/20477724.2017.1281374

Mol, A. (2008). *The logic of care: Health and the problem of patient choice.* Routledge.

Mole, B. (2017). Antivaccine groups step up work as Minnesota measles outbreak rages. *Ars Technica.* https://arstechnica.com/science/2017/06/anti-vaccine-groups-step-up-work-as-minnesota-measles-outbreak-rages/

Molteni, M. (2017). Anti-vaxxers brought their war to Minnesota—then came measles. *Wired.* https://www.wired.com/2017/05/anti-vaxxers-brought-war-minnesota-came-measles/

Molteni, M. (2020). What forest floor playgrounds teach us about kids and germs. *Wired.* https://www.wired.com/story/what-forest-floor-playgrounds-teach-us-about-kids-and-germs/

Moro, P. L., Arana, J., Marquez, P. L., Ng, C., Barash, F., Hibbs, B. F., & Cano, M. (2019). Is there any harm in administering extra-doses of vaccine to a person? Excess doses of vaccine reported to the vaccine adverse event reporting system (VAERS), 2007–2017. *Vaccine, 37*(28), 3730–3734. https://doi.org/10.1016/j.vaccine.2019.04.088

Mulcahy, E. R., Buchheit, C., Max, E., Hawley, S. R., & James, A. S. (2019). Collaborative health education for Somali Bantu refugee women in Kansas City. *BMC research notes, 12*(1), 616. https://doi.org/10.1186/s13104-019-4649-6

Mulle, J. G., Sharp, W. G., & Cubells, J. F. (2013). The gut microbiome: A new frontier in autism research. *Current Psychiatry Reports, 15*(2) Article 337. https://doi.org/10.1007/s11920-012-0337-0

Mullen, P. D. (1997). Compliance becomes concordance. *British Medical Journal, 314*(7082), 691–692. https://doi.org/10.1136/bmj.314.7082.691

National Institutes of Health (NIH). (2021). Health Literacy. https://www.nih.gov/institutes-nih/nih-office-director/office-communications-public-liaison/clear-communication/health-literacy

Nazaryan, A. (2017). In Minnesota, a measles outbreak exposes the gaps in public health. Public Radio Exchange. https://theworld.org/stories/2017/05/18/minnesota-it-s-not-just-about-measles-it-s-about-filling-gaps-public-health

Nelson, A. (2011). *Body and soul: The Black Panther Party and the fight against medical discrimination.* University of Minnesota Press.

Newkirk, V. R. (2016). Precision medicine's post-racial promise. *The Atlantic.* https://www.theatlantic.com/politics/archive/2016/06/precision-medicine-race-future/486143/

NIH Human Microbiome Project. (2012). National Institutes of Health. https://hmpdacc.org/hmp/

Njeru, J. W., Patten, C. A., Hanza, M. M., Brockman, T. A., Ridgeway, J. L., Weis, J. A., Clark, M. M., Goodson, M., Osman, A., Porraz-Capetillo, G., Hared, A., Myers, A., Sia, I. G., & Wieland, M. L. (2015). Stories for change: Development of a diabetes digital storytelling intervention for refugees and immigrants to Minnesota using qualitative methods. *BMC Public Health, 15,* Article 1311. https://doi.org/10.1186/s12889-015-2628-y

Nowicki, J. M. (2018). *K–12 Education: Discipline disparities for Black Students, Boys, and students with disabilities.* Report to congressional requesters. GAO-18-258. US Government Accountability Office. https://www.gao.gov/products/gao-18-258

Nur, S. A. (2022). On being and becoming Black in a globally dispersed diaspora. *Rhetoric Society Quarterly, 52*(3), 257–269. https://doi.org/10.1080/02773945.2022.2077626

Office of Disease Prevention and Health Promotion. (2020). Healthy People 2030. US Department of Health and Human Services. https://odphp.health.gov/healthypeople

Oh, S. S., Galanter, J., Thakur, N., Pino-Yanes, M., Barcelo, N. E., White, M. J., de Bruin, D. M., Greenblatt, R. M., Bibbins-Domingo, K., Wu, A. H. B., Borrell, L. N., Gunter, C., Powe, N. R., & Burchard, E. G. (2015). Diversity in clinical and biomedical research: A promise yet to be fulfilled. *PLoS Medicine, 12*(12), Article e1001918. https://doi.org/10.1371/journal.pmed.1001918

Ohayon, J. L., Cordner, A., Amico, A., Brown, P., & Richter, L. (2023). Persistent chemicals, persistent activism: Scientific opportunity structures and social movement organizing on contamination by per-and polyfluoroalkyl substances. *Social Movement Studies, ahead-of-print*, 1–23. https://doi.org/10.1080/14742837.2023.2178403

Orsini, M., & Smith, M. (2010). Social movements, knowledge and public policy: The case of autism activism in Canada and the US. *Critical Policy Studies, 4*(1), 38–57. https://doi.org/10.1080/19460171003714989

Owens, K. H. (2013). *Writing childbirth: Women's rhetorical agency in labor and online.* Southern Illinois Press.

Partinen, M., Saarenpää-Heikkilä, O., Ilveskoski, I., Hublin, C., Linna, M., Olsén, P., Nokelainen, P., Alén, R., Wallden, T., Espo, M., Rusanen, H., Olme, J., Sätilä, H., Arikka, H., Kaipainen, P., Julkunen, I., & Kirjavainen, T. (2012). Increased incidence and clinical picture of childhood narcolepsy following the 2009 H1N1 pandemic vaccination campaign in Finland. *PloS One, 7*(3), Article e33723. https://doi.org/10.1371/journal.pone.0033723

Paxson, H. (2012). *The life of cheese: The making of food and value in America.* University of California Press.

Pengilly, C. (2020). Rhetorics of empowerment for managing lupus pain: Patient-to-patient knowledge sharing in online health forums. In J. White-Farnham, B. Siegel Finer, & C. Molloy (Eds.), *Women's health advocacy: Rhetorical ingenuity for the 21st Century* (pp. 45–58). Routledge.

Pollan, M. (2013). Some of my best friends are germs. *New York Times Magazine.* https://www.nytimes.com/2013/05/19/magazine/say-hello-to-the-100-trillion-bacteria-that-make-up-your-microbiome.html?ref=magazine

Rapp, R. (1999). *Testing women, testing the fetus: The social impact of amniocentesis in America.* Routledge.

Ratcliffe, K. (2005). *Rhetorical listening: Identification, gender, whiteness.* Southern Illinois University Press.

Ravel, J., and Brotman, R. M. (2016). Translating the vaginal microbiome: Gaps and challenges. *Genome Medicine, 8*(35), 35. https://doi.org/10.1186/s13073-016-0291-2

Rees, G., & Gilman, N. (2018). Microbes are us: Let's not ignore this crisis any longer. *Washington Post.* https://www.washingtonpost.com/news/theworldpost/wp/2018/02/26/microbes/

Reich, J. A. (2014). Neoliberal mothering and vaccine refusal: Imagined gated communities and the privilege of choice. *Gender & Society, 28*(5), 679–704. https://doi.org/10.1177/0891243214532711

Reich, J. A. (2016). *Calling the shots: Why parents reject vaccines.* New York University Press.

Richert, C. (2018). A year after severe outbreak, more Somali American kids are vaccinated against the measles. *NPR News.* https://www.mprnews.org/story/2018/08/24/measles-vaccinated-somali-american-children-up-more-outbreak

Roberts, D. (1997). *Killing the Black body: Race, reproduction, and the meaning of liberty.* Penguin.

Roberts, D. (2001). *Shattered bonds: The color of child welfare.* Civitas Books.

Roberts, D. (2011). *Fatal invention: How science, politics, and big business re-create race in the twenty-first century.* New Press.

Roberts, D. (2022). *Torn apart: How the child welfare system destroys Black families—and abolition can build a safer world*. Basic Books.

Rook, G. A. (2012). Hygiene hypothesis and autoimmune diseases. *Clinical Reviews in Allergy & Immunology, 42*(1), 5–15. https://doi.org/10.1007/s12016-011-8285-8

Samudzi, Z. (2017). We need to talk about anti-vaxxing in Black communities. *Afropunk*. https://afropunk.com/2017/07/need-talk-anti-vaxxing-black-communities/

Schuster, M. (2006). A different place to birth: A material rhetoric analysis of BabyHaven, a freestanding birth center. *Women's Studies in Communication, 29*(1), 1–38. https://doi.org/10.1080/07491409.2006.10757626

schuster, s. (2021). *Trans medicine: The emergence and practice of treating gender*. New York University Press.

Scott, J. B. (2003). *Risky rhetoric: AIDS and the cultural practices of HIV testing*. Southern Illinois University Press.

Segal, J. Z. (2005). *Health and the rhetoric of medicine*. Southern Illinois University Press.

Shepherd S. M. (2018). Cultural awareness training for health professionals may have unintended consequences. *BMJ Opinion*. http://blogs.bmj.com/bmj/2018/01/22/stephane-m-shepherd-cultural-awareness-training-for-health-professionals-can-have-unintended-consequences

Shepherd, S. M. (2019). Cultural awareness workshops: Limitations and practical consequences. *BMC Medical Education, 19*(1), 14. https://doi.org/10.1186/s12909-018-1450-5

Shukla, S., Rastogi, S., Abdi, S. A. H., Dhamija, P., Kumar, V., Kalaiselvan, V., & Medhi, B. (2021). Severe cutaneous adverse reactions in Asians: Trends observed in culprit anti-seizure medicines using VigiBase®. *Seizure, 91*, 332–338. https://doi.org/10.1016/j.seizure.2021.07.011

Silverman, C. (2012). *Understanding autism: Parents, doctors, and the history of a disorder*. Princeton University Press.

Simpson, A. (2007). On ethnographic refusal: Indigeneity, "voice" and colonial citizenship. *Junctures: The Journal for Thematic Dialogue, 9*, 67–80.

Simpson, A. (2014). *Mohawk interruptus: Political life across the borders of settler states*. Duke University Press.

Simpson, A. (2017). The ruse of consent and the anatomy of "refusal": Cases from Indigenous North America and Australia. *Postcolonial Studies, 20*(1), 18–33.

Skiba, R. J., Michael, R. S., Nardo, A. C., & Peterson, R. L. (2002). The color of discipline: Sources of racial and gender disproportionality in school punishment. *The Urban Review, 34*(4), 317–342. https://doi.org/10.1023/A:1021320817372

Skinner, D., & Franz, B. (2018). From patients to populations: Rhetorical considerations for a post-compliance medicine. *Rhetoric of Health & Medicine, 1*(3), 239–268. https://doi.org/10.5744/rhm.2018.1013

Smedley, B. D., Stith, A. Y., Evans, C. H., Colburn, L., Association of American Medical Colleges, Institute of Medicine, & Association of Academic Health Centers. (2001). *The right thing to do, the smart thing to do: Enhancing diversity in the health professions—summary of the symposium on diversity in health professions*. National Academies Press. https://doi.org/10.17226/10186

Smilges, J. L. (2022). *Queer Silence: On disability and rhetorical absence*. University of Minnesota Press.

Snyder, J. E., Upton, R. D., Hassett, T. C., Lee, H., Nouri, Z., & Dill, M. (2023). Black representation in the primary care physician workforce and its association with population life expectancy and mortality rates in the US. *JAMA Network Open, 6*(4), Article e236687. https://doi.org/10.1001/jamanetworkopen.2023.6687

Sobo, E. J. (2015). Social cultivation of vaccine refusal and delay among Waldorf school parents: Social cultivation of vaccine refusal. *Medical Anthropology Quarterly, 29*(3), 381–399. https://doi.org/10.1111/maq.12214

Sobo, E. J. (2016). Theorizing (vaccine) refusal: Through the looking glass. *Cultural Anthropology, 31*(3), 342–350. https://doi.org/10.14506/ca31.3.04

Sohn, E. (2017). Understanding the history behind communities' vaccine fears. *NPR*. https://www.npr.org/sections/health-shots/2017/05/03/526595475/understanding-the-history-behind-communities-vaccine-fears

Somalis in Minnesota Oral History Project. (2016). Minnesota Historical Society. http://www2.mnhs.org/library/findaids/oh176.xml

Stallins, J. A., Law, D. M., Strosberg, S. A., & Rossi, J. J. (2018). Geography and postgenomics: how space and place are the new DNA. *GeoJournal, 83*(1), 153–168. http://www.jstor.org/stable/45117486

Strachan, D. P. (1989). Hay fever, hygiene, and household size. *BMJ, 299*(6710), 1259–1260. https://doi.org/10.1136/bmj.299.6710.1259

Sun, L. (2017). Antivaccine activists spark a state's worst measles outbreak in decades. *Washington Post*. https://www.washingtonpost.com/national/health-science/antivaccine-activists-spark-a-states-worst-measles-outbreak-in-decades/2017/05/04/a1fac952-2f39-11e7-9dec-764dc781686f_story.html?utm_term=.1d4948cd39ca

Sunni, M., Kyllo, J., Brunzell, C., Majcozak, J., Osman, M., Dhunkal, A. M., & Moran, A. (2023). A picture is worth a thousand words: A culturally-tailored video-based approach to diabetes education in Somali families of children with type 1 diabetes. *Journal of Clinical & Translational Endocrinology, 31*, Article 100313. https://doi.org/10.1016/j.jcte.2023.100313

Swartz, A. (2017). "Anti-vaxxers 'targeted' Minnesota's Somali community: Now they have a measles outbreak." *Mic*. https://www.mic.com/articles/174489/anti-vaxxers-targeted-minnesota-s-somali-community-now-they-have-a-measles-outbreak

Taylor, D. E. (2014). *Toxic communities: Environmental racism, industrial pollution, and residential mobility*. New York University Press.

Tervalon, M., & Murray-García, J. (1998). Cultural humility versus cultural competence: A critical distinction in defining physician training outcomes in multicultural education. *Journal of Health Care for the Poor and Underserved, 9*(2), 117–125. https://doi.org/10.1353/hpu.2010.0233

Teston, C. (2024). *Doing dignity: Ethical praxis and the politics of care*. Johns Hopkins University Press.

Thornton, C., & Reich, J. A. (2022). Black mothers and vaccine refusal: Gendered racism, healthcare, and the state. *Gender & Society, 36*(4), 525–551. https://doi.org/10.1177/08912432221102150

Toh, M., & Allen-Vercoe, E. (2015). The human gut microbiota with reference to autism spectrum disorder: Considering the whole as more than a sum of its parts. *Microbial Ecology in Health and Disease, 26*(1), 263–279. https://doi.org/10.3402/mehd.v26.26309

Trostle, J. A. (1988). Medical compliance as an ideology. *Social Science and Medicine, 27*(12), 1299–1308.

Trostle, J. A. (1997). The history and meaning of patient compliance as an ideology. In D. S. Gochman (Ed.), *Handbook of health behavior research II* (pp. 109–124). Springer.

Tuck, E., & Yang, K. W. (2014a). R-words: Refusing research. In D. Paris & M. T. Winn (Eds.), *Humanizing research: Decolonizing qualitative Inquiry with Youth and Communities* (pp. 223–247). Sage Publications.

Tuck, E., & Yang, K. W. (2014b). Unbecoming claims: Pedagogies of refusal in qualitative research. *Qualitative inquiry, 20*(6), 811–818. https://doi.org/10.1177/1077800414530265

Ursell, L. K., Metcalf, J. L., Parfrey, L. W., & Knight, R. (2012). Defining the human microbiome. *Nutrition Reviews, 70*(8), S38–S44. https://doi.org/10.1111/j.1753-4887.2012.00493.x

US Department of Education Office for Civil Rights. (2014). Civil rights data collection, data snapshot: School discipline. https://civilrightsdata.ed.gov/assets/downloads/2011-12_CRDC-School-Discipline-Snapshot.pdf

Vangay, P., Johnson, A. J., Ward, T. L., Al-Ghalith, G. A., Shields-Cutler, R. R., Hillmann, B. M., Lucas, S. K., Beura, L. K., Thompson, E. A., Till, L. M., Batres, R., Paw, B., Pergament, S. L., Saenyakul, P., Xiong, M., Kim, A. D., Kim, G., Masopust, D., Martens, E. C., Angkurawaranon, C., . . . Knights, D. (2018). US immigration westernizes the human gut microbiome. *Cell, 175*(4), 962–972.e10. https://doi.org/10.1016/j.cell.2018.10.029

Velasquez-Manoff, M. (2012). *An epidemic of absence: A new way of understanding allergies and autoimmune diseases.* Scribner.

Villarosa, L. (2023). *Under the skin: The hidden toll of racism on health in America.* Penguin.

Vinson, J. (2017). *Embodying the problem: The persuasive power of the teen mother.* Rutgers University Press.

Vogel, G. (2015). Why a pandemic flu shot caused narcolepsy. *Science.* https://www.science.org/content/article/why-pandemic-flu-shot-caused-narcolepsyhttps://www.science.org/content/article/why-pandemic-flu-shot-caused-narcolepsy

Voyles, T. B. (2020). Green lovin' mamas don't vax! The pseudo-environmentalism of anti-vaccination discourse. *Studies in the Humanities, 46*(1–2). https://doi.org/10.1177/136346150003700306

Wagner, J. (2017). Vaccines challenged at Twin Cities measles meeting. *CBS.* http://minnesota.cbslocal.com/2017/04/30/vaccine-safety-council-measles-outbreak/

Waite, G. (1987). Public health in pre-colonial East Central Africa. *Social Science and Medicine, 24*(3), 197–208. http://doi.org/10.1koerbo16/0277-9536(87)90047-5

Walters, S. (2014). *Rhetorical touch: Disability, identification, haptics.* University of South Carolina Press.

Weibel, D., Sturkenboom, M., Black, S., de Ridder, M., Dodd, C., Bonhoeffer, J., Vanrolleghem, A., van der Maas, N., Lammers, G. J., Overeem, S., Gentile, A., Giglio, N., Castellano, V., Kwong, J. C., Murray, B. J., Cauch-Dudek, K., Juhasz, D., Campitelli, M., Datta, A. N., Kallweit, U., Huang, W. T., Huang, Y. S., Hsu, C. Y., Chen, H. C., Giner-Soriano, M., Morros, R., Gaig, C., Tió E., Perez-Vilar, S., Diez-Domingo, J., Puertas, F. J., Svenson L. W., Mahmud, S. M., Carleton, B., Naus, M., Arnheim-Dahlström, L., Pedersen, L., DeStefano, F., & Shimabukuro, T. T. (2018). Narcolepsy and adjuvanted pandemic influenza A (H1N1) 2009 vaccines—Multi-country assessment. *Vaccine, 36*(41): 6202–6211. https://doi.org/10.1016/j.vaccine.2018.08.008

Welhausen, C. A., Popham, S. L., Kondrlik, K. E., Lawrence, H. Y., & Scott, J. L. (2015). Rhetoric, ebola, and vaccination: A conversation among scholars. *Poroi, 11*(2). https://doi.org/10.13008/2151-2957.1232

Wentzell, E., & Racila, A. (2021). The social experience of participation in a COVID-19 vaccine trial: Subjects' motivations, others' concerns, and insights for vaccine promotion. *Vaccine, 39*(17), 2445–2451. https://doi.org/10.1016/j.vaccine.2021.03.036

White, L. (2000). *Speaking with vampires: Rumor and history in colonial Africa.* University of California Press.

World Health Organization (WHO). (2019). Ten threats to global health in 2019. https://www.who.int/news-room/spotlight/ten-threats-to-global-health-in-2019

Wu, A. H., White, M. J., Oh, S., & Burchard, E. (2015). The Hawaii Clopidogrel lawsuit: The possible effect on clinical laboratory testing. *Personalized medicine, 12*(3), 179–181. https://doi.org/10.2217/pme.15.4

Yam, S. S. (2019). *Inconvenient strangers: Transnational subjects and the politics of citizenship*. The Ohio State University Press.

Yergeau, M. R. (2018). *Authoring autism: On rhetoric and neurological queerness*. Duke University Press.

Yong, E. (2016). *I contain multitudes: The microbes within us and a grander view of life*. HarperCollins.

Zarowsky, C. (2000). Trauma stories: Violence, emotion and politics in Somali Ethiopia. *Transcultural Psychiatry, 37*(3), 383–402. https://doi.org/10.1177/136346150003700306

Zavestoski, S., Brown, P., McCormick, S., Mayer, B., D'Ottavi, M., & Lucove, J. C. (2004). Patient activism and the struggle for diagnosis: Gulf war illnesses and other medically unexplained physical symptoms in the US. *Social Science & Medicine, 58*(1), 161–175. https://doi.org/10.1016/S0277-9536(03)00157-6

INDEX

Abdi, Cawo M., 112–13

ableism, 36–37, 43, 112, 143; and antivaccination, 37; and racism, 63–64, 67–70

adaptive: equipment, 134, 181; services, 118, 134

adherence, 9–10. *See also* compliance/noncompliance

adverse reactions, 89, 95, 99, 105

advocacy: and autism, 3–4, 72–74, 114–16; health, 19–20, 105–7. *See also* citizen science; mothers; parents

affect, 97, 109, 127, 159–63, 170–72, 175–76; and suspicion, 21–22

agency, 39, 79–82, 87; and choice, 119, 138, 141–45; and power, 28–30; rhetorical, 26–29

Allen-Vercoe, Emma, 151, 173

antibiotics, 89, 95, 97, 101, 151–52, 154, 157, 174, 177–79

antivaccination: campaigns, 3–4, 74–75, 82–84; frames used to cover, 79–81, 84–87; history of, 75–76; and mothers, 77–81, 84–87; and outbreak, 3–5, 37, 39, 82–87. *See also* science; vaccines; vaccine hesitancy

Applied Behavior Analysis (ABA) therapy, 47–49, 50, 116

arhetorical/nonrhetorical acts, 26, 27, 29, 78

autism, 1–2, 36–38; as diagnosis, 119–24, 160–62; discourses of, 55–72, 172, 179–81, 185; environmental theories of, 46, 98, 103, 152, 179; genetic theories of, 46, 66; in health literacy education, 44–49; and microbiome, 147, 152, 157, 165n2, 168, 177; and MMR vaccine, 72–75, 76–77, 82–86, 99; personal accounts of, 41, 52–53, 92, 97–98, 157–58, 174–75, 177–78; and race, 114–16; in social services, 110–12, 114–16, 124–41, 162–63; and Somali children, 3–4, 41–43, 82; and stigma, 37, 124. *See also* community sickness

Autism Self Advocacy Network (ASAN), 47

belief: and culture, 16; and dissent, 30; systems, 90, 93–94, 148; wrong, 41, 58, 74–81, 86–87, 99, 106, 128–29. *See also* depoliticization; individualism; vaccines

belonging/nonbelonging, 19, 54–55, 56–57, 59, 62–64, 74, 114–16, 119–24, 188; and refusal, 6, 24, 102–3, 148, 179–82, 188. *See also* citizenship; public good

Benezra, Amber, 154–56

Benjamin, Ruha, 17, 23–24, 80, 147, 187

biomedical: approaches to autism, 36, 43, 55, 56, 124, 126, 129–30, 135, 142–43, 145, 171–72, 189; approaches to disability, 20, 55; approaches to vaccination, 11, 21, 78, 156; authority, 11, 18, 190; colonialism, 14; knowledge production, 105, 173; racism, 80, 155, 187. *See also* evidence-based medicine; medicine; medicalization

biosocial group, 19, 54, 96, 119, 123, 148, 165n2, 180

biotechnologies, 13–14, 109. *See also* vaccines

Biss, Eula, 80n1

Black feminist theory, 20

Blackness, 60–61; colonial management of, 14, 21n4, 155; and/in medicine, 80, 108, 154; and racism, 59, 69, 127, 128; and rhetorical agency, 28; and vaccines, 80, 80n1

Blaser, Martin, 152, 154

bodies: and affect, 21–22; knowledge from, 55, 65–66, 88–91, 95–99, 104–8, 173–76; and/as microbiome, 150–56; standard, 8–9, 40, 45–49, 189; and vaccination, 93–94, 142–45

breastfeeding, 154

Brown, Phil, 106

capitalism: and care, 94–96, 137–41; and colonialism, 21; and disability, 20; and disease, 95n4, 102–3, 177; and microbiome, 148–49, 155; and refugee resettlement, 112–14; and vaccination, 94–96, 95n4, 102–3

care, 21–22, 31, 40, 43–44, 69, 93–96, 120, 123–24; and caregiving labor, 137–41; in health systems, 44–45, 168; inequities in, 83–84, 97, 99, 132–33; and/as language, 141; and/for microbiome, 147, 152–53, 168–70, 174, 178–79; practices of, 58, 71, 89, 93–96, 163–65, 166–68; and/as refusal, 91–103, 109, 135–36, 143–46; and reporting, 137–40; and/in social services, 116–19, 130–31, 137–39, 142

case managers, 117–18, 131, 138, 159–61, 169, 173

Centers for Disease Control and Prevention (CDC), 12, 105

cesarean birth, 97, 151, 154, 157

Charles, Nicole, 11, 13, 21–22, 21n4, 80, 97n5, 187

child protective services, 80, 127. *See also* surveillance

childbirth, 97, 151, 154, 157, 169–70

childcare, 2n1, 85, 86, 95, 137–40, 153

citizen science, 65–66, 105–6. *See also* expertise

citizenship, 127; health, 18, 95–96, 105–7, 156. *See also* belonging/nonbelonging

Clare, Eli, 143

class, 28, 81; and autism, 132; and microbiome, 153–54, 157; and vaccination, 77–78, 87

climate, 1, 53, 65, 98, 103

clinical trials, 91–92, 103–8, 115, 174; and race, 104–5, 107–8. *See also* knowledge; science

clinics, 168–69, 170–72

collectivity, 37, 40, 68, 70, 179; and activism, 58–61, 68, 176, 177, 185, 190; and care, 67, 123, 135, 143, 176, 180

colonialism: and disability, 20; and medical research, 155–56; and microbiome, 150–52, 154–56; and refusal, 23; and vaccines, 13–14, 18, 92n3

community health workers, 25, 57, 120, 124, 125, 133, 137, 168, 180

community sickness (term), 36–37, 38, 40, 42–43, 98, 100–108, 123–24, 136, 147, 148, 157, 178–79, 180–81, 185, 188–90; discourses of, 52–68; as fertile ground, 70–71

compliance/noncompliance, 7–10, 11–12, 17, 25–26, 31, 85; and vaccines, 102, 109, 186–87

concordance, 9–10. *See also* compliance/noncompliance

Conis, Elena, 75–77

consent, 9, 23

consumer-directed care, 116–17, 139

contributory expertise (term), 65, 104, 108. *See also* citizen science

counterstory (term), 34, 65, 130, 141

criminalization, 58, 127, 189. *See also* child protective services; police

critical disability studies, 20, 36–37. *See also* collectivity; disability culture, 57, 60–61, 113, 136, 186; as frame, 14–16, 85, 106; and health outcomes, 14–15; and social services, 127–28; and trainings, 9, 14–16

cures: and autism, 41, 58, 128–29; and disability, 20

Decoteau, Clare L. 67, 79, 115–16, 132, 165n2

deficit-based: approaches to literacy, 11, 13, 18; solutions, 84–85; understandings of autism, 43, 55, 56, 124, 126, 129–30, 135, 142–43, 145, 171–72, 189; understandings of science, 6

denial of services, 111, 130, 131, 132, 133, 141, 168

dependence, 125, 130, 143, 145; pathologized, 136. *See also* collectivity; independence; interdependence

depoliticization, 68, 102, 155–57. *See also* neoliberalism

Derkatch, Colleen, 173–74

developmental disabilities, 24, 43, 47, 73–74, 99, 121, 133

diagnosis, 36, 41–42, 60, 62, 63, 67, 68, 69, 112, 114, 118, 119–24, 127–29, 143, 160–61, 163, 181; and rates of autism, 73

diaspora, 3, 38, 41, 111–14; African, 60–61; and autism, 52, 54, 58, 63–65, 67–71, 178, 189; and family, 144. *See also* migration; Somalis

diet: and autism, 48–49, 64, 115; and microbiome, 40, 147, 149, 151–54, 157, 164, 167–68, 170, 172, 174, 176, 181, 185; and migration, 98, 103. *See also* food; microbiome

dirt, 93, 149, 153, 156

disability, 20, 36–37; medical model of, 43, 55, 56, 124, 126, 129–30, 135, 142–43, 145, 171–72, 189; social model of, 54, 56–58, 61, 67, 180

disclosure, 112, 124–27. *See also* deficit-based

disease, 7–9, 89; and autism, 59; control of, 78, 93, 95–96, 102, 156; and/in microbiome, 150, 151–52, 156–57, 172–73; and race and ethnicity, 104–5, 93; outbreak, 3, 74, 82–83, 88; and risk, 11, 90–91; as vaccine-preventable, 76, 78, 99

disease cluster, 3, 41, 64–65, 73, 106, 114

disinformation, 4, 5, 6, 43, 70, 82, 83, 84, 85, 86

Disneyland, 77–78

"Do not resuscitate" (DNR) worksheet, 142

doctors: and authority, 170; dismissal by, 97, 121; engagement with, 45–47, 52–53, 122, 163, 171–72; and patient compliance, 8; perceptions of, 89, 181; and pharmaceuticals, 166; trust in, 171–72. *See also* biomedical; care; medicine

Dolmage, Jay T., 26

Dorpenyo, Isidore K., 14

dysbiosis, 151, 175. *See also* microbiome

early interventions, 115

education: and cultural competence, 15, 141; and literacy, 13–14; and noncompliance, 141; and/in refugee resettlement, 113–14; and Somali youth, 69, 74, 132, 136; and vaccine hesitancy, 21n4, 67, 79, 83, 85–86, 186. *See also* literacy

embodiment: and knowledge, 55, 65–66, 88–92, 96–99, 173–76; and trauma, 5, 174–76. *See also* bodies; contributory expertise; evidence; expertise

environmental racism, 65, 98, 103

environment-caused illness, 65, 106, 180

epidemics of absence (term), 152. *See also* dysbiosis; microbiome

epistemic marginalization (term), 169, 188. *See also* agency; rhetoric; rhetorical refusal; silence

Epstein, Stephen, 107–8

eradication, 78–79, 95, 102–3

ethos, 26–29, 34, 78, 188

evictions, 63, 69–70. *See also* housing

evidence, 90, 173–74, 182–84; and autism, 119–24, 131; contestations of, 89, 91, 103–8; and microbiome, 175–76; and/for social services, 141, 144–45. *See also* biomedical; embodiment; science

evidence-based medicine, 43, 48–49, 146, 173–74, 182–85, 187; and autism, 115–16; and clinical trials, 103–8; and race, 17, 91–92; and vaccination, 90–99. *See also* biomedical; evidence; medicine

exigence, 43, 70, 80, 100, 102; material, 102. *See also* fertile ground

experimental remedies, 131, 147, 157, 166, 181

expertise, 14, 16, 19, 21, 26, 106, 108, 170, 183, 184; and/through disability, 135, 142; dis/trust in, 65; and ethos, 27; lived, 65, 103, 167; and vaccination, 79, 83, 87, 91, 99, 104

family, 4, 6, 55–56, 58, 63, 69–70, 126, 132, 144; in resettlement, 113; state evaluations of, 111–12, 118, 124–25, 129, 133–35, 139, 143. See also diaspora; mothers; parents

family separation, 127–30, 176

fertile ground (term), 5, 30–31, 38, 43, 55, 66, 70–71, 83, 147, 184, 190. See also exigence; rhetorical refusal

Fisher, Jill A., 107–8

flexible immunity (term), 93–94

flu vaccine, 76, 105

food: and access, 69, 98–99, 102, 132, 136, 144, 175; and class, 77; and culture, 61, 98; deserts, 30; and family, 61, 167, 171; and microbiome, 149, 152, 153, 163, 166–68, 169, 174, 178, 180; and migration, 53, 65, 66, 157; in refugee resettlement, 113, 175; and vaccination, 53, 65, 66, 77, 98. See also diet; microbiome

Fricker, Miranda, 27

futurity, 23, 25, 27, 29–31, 34–35, 38, 40, 55, 88, 143, 147–48, 158, 176, 179–82, 184, 188

gastrointestinal disorders, 46, 48, 52, 97, 164. See also diet; microbiome

gender: and authority, 28; and/in clinical trials, 107; and microbiome, 40, 154–55; and race, 59, 81; and/in refugee resettlement, 113; and vaccination, 74, 75, 77–80. See also ethos; mothers; race

Glabau, Donya, 106

global South, 18, 80–81, 152, 155

Goldenberg, Maya, 16–17, 182–83

Gouge, Catherine, 8–9, 26

government distrust, 16–17, 96–99, 113, 163

Greene, Jeremy A., 7–8

gut feelings, 97, 109, 127, 175–76

Happe, Kelly E., 155, 180

Harper, Kimberly C., 28

Hausman, Bernice L., 5, 17, 34, 78–79, 80n1, 93, 95n4, 98, 183

healthcare, 31–33, 169; agency within, 166, 167, 176; and cost, 4, 99, 102, 123; critiques of, 19–20, 141; and culture, 14–16, 141; and discrimination, 97, 101, 103; education about, 24, 43–46; for microbiome, 147, 168, 179; neoliberalization of, 113–15, 138; and policy, 113–15, 154; and racism, 97; in refugee resettlement, 42, 81, 103, 123; rejection of, 6–10, 30–31; in Somalia, 89, 92n3, 93; and specialization, 114, 132; and trust, 16–18, 172; and vaccines, 9, 76, 79, 85. See also biomedical; medicine; public health

health disparities, 83, 105, 149, 154–55, 157, 177, 185

health insurance, 13, 97, 115, 181

health literacy, 2–14, 24–25, 30, 31, 38, 42–54, 66–68, 70, 79, 89, 92, 103, 110, 129, 141, 145, 171, 178, 187, 188; curriculum, 44–47, 56, 57

health outcomes, 13, 15

healthy community, 102

Healthy People 2030, 12

helminthic therapy, 152–53

hepatitis B vaccine, 76, 91

herbal remedies, 165

herd immunity, 100–101

hesitancy, 10–11. See also vaccine hesitancy

Hib, 105

home visits, 162–63, 169, 172, 173

housing, 43, 62–64, 69, 70, 98, 99, 101, 102, 113, 136, 144, 180, 181

HPV vaccine, 13, 21

hygiene hypothesis, 151

immigrants: and vaccines, 81–84; and vulnerability, 81, 82. See also migration; race; refugees

immunity, 78, 85, 92n3, 93–94. See also vaccines

independence, 130–36, 142–43, 145

individualism, 136, 138, 140, 148, 150–52, 156; and health decision-making, 10; and parenting, 55

infectious diseases: and outbreak, 3, 74, 82–83, 88–89; and risk, 11, 77–78, 89, 90–91; and vaccines, 76–78, 99 institutional documents: application processes, 117–19; and bureaucratic writing, 110–12, 119–21

insurance. *See* health insurance

intellectual disabilities, 73. *See also* autism; disability

interdependence, 143, 184. *See also* collectivity; dependence

interpreters, 4, 84, 85

interviews, 31–35

Islam, 103, 132, 185

Islamophobia, 64, 103, 185

Jack, Jordynn, 78

Kafer, Alison, 20

Keränen, Lisa, 136, 142

knowledge: contestations of, 27–28, 173–75; embodied, 55, 65–66, 88–91, 95–99, 104–8, 173–76; subjugated, 14, 27–29, 169–70. *See also* ethos; evidence; science

Lawrence, Heidi Y., 77, 93, 102

Lay, Mary, 28

Linton, Simi, 36

listening, 26–31, 34, 40, 66, 108, 182–84, 189–90. *See also* fertile ground; rhetorical listening; rhetorical refusal

literacy: bureaucratic, 80, 112, 179; class, 5, 24–25, 31–32, 38, 43–52, 54, 56–57, 70, 110, 171, 180, 188, 189; English language, 113, 145; as frame, 16, 18, 26, 42, 66, 70, 103, 106, 141; health, 7, 10–11, 12–14, 30–31, 66–68, 70, 79, 89, 129, 141, 145, 179, 187–89; scientific, 6, 31, 83–85, 129, 179

logic of care (term), 144

Lorimer, Jamie, 151, 153

mandates, 78–79, 93, 102, 187

Martin, Emily, 93

Martinez, Aja, 34, 34n6

measles: and outbreak, 2–5, 31, 39, 72, 77, 81, 82–87, 88, 91, 108, 110, 186; and risk, 99; in Somalia, 88–89. *See also* measles-mumps-rubella (MMR) vaccine; vaccines

measles-mumps-rubella (MMR) vaccine, 2–5, 24–25, 63, 65, 76, 78, 83; and autism, 76–77, 80; and Somali children, 2, 72, 76, 84–85; Somali participant accounts of, 2, 5, 90–92, 99

media: and methods, 32, 34; and/about microbiome, 149, 150–51; and/about Somalis, 3–5, 82–84, 84–87; and/about vaccination controversy, 3, 39, 72, 74–75, 76–77, 78–82, 83–84, 85–87

medical records, 79, 92, 92n3, 121, 123, 129, 168. *See also* diagnosis; silence; writing

medical testing, 107, 115, 159–61, 171, 173. *See also* autism; diagnosis; evidence

medicalization, 9, 20, 56, 68, 70, 115, 120, 130–37, 141–43, 154, 156, 169–70, 182–83, 187

medicine: alternative, 77, 131, 148, 162–65, 166–68; anxieties about, 74, 78, 94, 99; authority within, 78, 128; and autism, 112, 114–16, 119–24, 132–35, 158; and colonialism, 80–81, 153–56; critiques of, 142; distrust of, 78, 96, 98; and diversity, 15, 96–98, 103–5, 107; evidence within, 89, 90–91, 103, 106–7, 131; and microbiome, 153–56, 166–68; personalized, 93, 149–50; and racism, 75, 80, 96–97, 104, 153–56; rejections of, 77–78, 144, 147–48; Western, 95, 104, 108, 130. *See also* biomedical; doctors; evidence-based medicine; healthcare; vaccines

microbiome: and autism, 5, 37; diversity of, 149–50, 151–52, 152–53; and gender, 153–54; infantile development of, 152, 154; media coverage of/and, 148, 149–51; and migration, 152, 175, 177; and race, 155–56; and research, 155; and rhetorical refusal, 40, 67, 147, 179–82; and Somali mothers, 32, 148, 157, 163–65, 166, 169, 170, 173–76, 178; and wellness industry, 149, 157

migration: and microbiome, 152, 157, 165n2, 174, 177; reverse, 58; and Somali refugees, 2n2, 4, 37–39, 49, 59, 64, 66, 68, 69, 88, 92–93, 94, 101, 103, 112–13, 173, 176, 178, 180, 185; vaccination during, 92

milestones, developmental, 25, 47, 49, 50

Minneapolis, 1, 2–4, 2n2, 31, 72–73, 84, 94, 158

Minneapolis Somali Autism Spectrum Disorder Prevalence Project, 3, 72–73

Minnesota, 1, 13, 31, 44, 52, 58, 59, 61, 67, 72, 94, 157, 170, 174, 177, 186; and measles outbreak, 2–5, 72–73, 81, 82–88, 108, 189

Minnesota Department of Health (MDH), 2, 2n1, 4, 5, 72, 84–86

misinformation. *See* disinformation

Mol, Annemarie, 138, 172, 184

mothers: and activism, 106, 114–16, 165n2; and autism, 61–62, 114–16; and caregiving, 38, 40, 55, 95, 123, 136, 143–44, 147, 167, 169, 179; and gender roles, 113; and health responsibility, 17–18, 154; and protection, 96, 98, 124, 188; and racism, 21, 28, 59, 60, 62, 75, 80n1, 126–27, 130; and surveillance, 80, 124, 126–27, 129, 130; and vaccination, 21, 74, 75, 77–82, 86–87. *See also* care; gender; parents; protection

National Institutes of Health (NIH), 12, 104, 150

naturopaths, 5, 32–33, 37, 40, 147, 163–65, 168, 169, 170–72, 173, 174, 179, 189

neoliberalism, 18, 22, 111, 115, 143, 156, 185. *See also* independence; individualism

neurodiversity, 36

neutrality: and ableism, 20, 112; and documentation, 111; and medicine, 10, 20; and science, 155; as stance in vaccination research, 34–35; and/used by the state, 111, 127, 189; and vaccines, 102; and whiteness, 116, 128

Nur, Suban Cooley, 60–61

nutrition. *See* diet; food; microbiome

Pandemrix, 105

parent responsibility factor (term), 133–34

parents: advocacy by, 3–4, 106, 165n2; beliefs of, 55–56, 63, 64–65, 88–89, 91, 93–94, 98, 99, 163; denial by, 162–63; as experts, 106, 167–69, 176; fears of, 59–60, 63, 90, 99–100, 127, 127–29; hopes of, 1–2, 59, 66, 69–70, 123, 128, 132, 133–34, 143–44, 145, 161, 164, 179, 184, 188; and race, 59–60, 61–62, 79–80, 87, 115–16, 132–33; and responsibility, 17–18, 131, 134, 154; and schools, 59–60, 122–23, 127–29, 161, 164; and social services, 113–14, 125, 131–35, 139, 143; surveillance of, 80, 124, 126–27, 129, 130, 160, 163; and vaccines, 77–81, 84–87, 90, 92, 95. *See also* mothers

personal belief exemption, 24, 77–80. *See also* antivaccination; belief; vaccine hesitancy; vaccines

personal care assistant or associate (PCA), 50, 57, 111, 117, 127

person-centered care, 116–17, 139

pharmaceuticals: and autism, 48, 166–67; and compliance, 8; critiques of, 19, 21–22, 65, 68, 89, 104–8; industry, 11, 21, 107, 187; trials and testing of, 14, 104–8; and vaccine hesitancy, 65, 76, 78. *See also* biomedical; medicalization; medicine

physicians. *See* doctors

Plavix, 105

police, 58, 59, 60, 127, 185. *See also* child protective services

policy: and clinical trials, 107; and disability, 114, 131, 139–40; health, 17, 18, 19, 78, 92, 101, 182, 188–89; vaccine, 78, 102

Pollan, Michael, 151, 152, 167

pollution, 53, 99, 175, 177; and vaccines, 37, 98. *See also* environmental racism; environment-caused illness

post-traumatic stress disorder (PTSD), 68

power: and activism, 20–21, 106, 114–15; and disability, 20, 114–15; and language, 36, 128; and medicine, 18, 28–29, 68, 74, 97, 104–9, 174, 183, 184; and research, 35; and rhetoric, 26–31, 79, 86–87; and rhetorical refusal, 6, 26, 29, 70, 81–82, 109, 140; and the state, 98–99, 115, 127, 130, 188; and vaccines, 81, 86–87

protection: of children, 90, 96, 98, 124, 188; rhetorical refusal and/as, 6, 25–26, 30, 40, 43, 71, 88, 91, 101, 188; state valuations of, 140; vaccines and/as, 6; vaccine refusal and/as, 22, 90, 92–93, 94, 96–97, 99–100, 109. *See also* rhetorical refusal

public assistance, 113–14, 117–19

public good, 78, 100–101

public health: distrust of, 24, 25, 71, 80, 83, 89, 91, 92, 96, 108, 148; global, 13–14, 21–22, 81; and inequalities, 14, 81, 101, 107; and methods, 31–33, 32n5; and outbreak, 3–4, 5, 19, 39, 72, 74, 83, 84–88, 109, 189; and vaccines, 11, 18, 41, 76, 79–80, 90, 92n3, 102, 178, 186

queer silence (term), 29

race: and autism, 2n1, 37, 61–62, 73–74, 114–15; in clinical research and testing, 91–93,

96–97, 103–8, 109, 154–56; Critical Race Theory, 34n6; definitions of, 104, 155; discrimination and, 60–62, 63; and health disparities, 19, 38, 43, 98, 105, 109, 155–56; and marginalization, 28, 61, 67, 70, 81, 96, 97–99, 115, 132; and medicine, 16, 17, 80, 150, 153, 155, 185, 187; and positionality, 35; and school, 96, 99, 101, 122–23, 126, 128–29; and surveillance, 70, 80, 124, 126–27, 129, 130, 145, 160, 163; and vaccines, 17, 75, 77–82, 90–93

racialization, 39, 58–62, 94, 104, 155

racism: accretive, 38, 43, 59, 67, 70, 156, 177; and autism, 43, 59, 61, 62, 64, 70, 129, 178; environmental, 17, 60–63, 98, 177; medical, 16, 17, 19, 38, 43, 65, 75, 80, 96–97, 98–99, 101, 103, 104–5, 109, 115, 150, 154, 155–56, 185, 187; and housing, 63; and school, 60, 70, 96, 99, 101, 122–23, 126, 128–29; and science, 17, 155, 185; and the state, 63, 70, 80, 96, 127, 129, 130, 145, 160, 163; systemic, 62–63, 67, 75, 154, 155, 177, 178, 185; and vaccine dissent, 75, 80, 88, 96, 100

Ratcliffe, Krista, 34n7, 183

refugees: and autism, 37; and health, 38, 64, 90–93, 94, 177–79; and precarity, 28, 38, 43, 59, 67, 70, 96–99, 113–14, 125–29, 175–76; resettlement of, 112–14. *See also* diaspora; migration; race; Somalis

refusal: affiliative, 24; ethnographic, 22–23; as frame, 22–24; informed, 23–24. *See also* rhetorical refusal

resistance, 19–21. *See also* refusal

respite care, 118, 133, 137

responsibility: and parenting, 45, 87, 131, 132, 134, 154; patient, 154, 187; personal, 70, 156, 185; shared, 140; and trust, 16; and vaccination, 96, 101

return migration, 58

Revitalization Act, 104

rhetoric: defined, 26–27; modes of, 26, 27, 28, 29, 122; and noncompliance, 26; and persuasion, 184; and power, 140

rhetorical listening, 29, 34n7, 183

rhetorical refusal: analysis of, 30–31, 148, 166, 182, 184, 185–87; and/through care, 40, 147, 179; defined, 5–8, 24–31; and/through documentation, 39, 112, 119, 120, 124, 129–31, 140–44; and/through embodiment, 39, 108; and epistemic value, 106–8; and/through language, 43, 70; and meaning-making, 28–29; modes of, 26–28; and protection, 101; and power, 5–6, 26–29, 71; and/as vaccine dissent, 75, 87, 88

rhetorical subjectivity, 77–81, 86–87

rhetoricity, 26, 27, 28, 29, 100, 144, 182

risk: and health activism, 103–8; management of, 97, 99, 156; and medicine, 9, 104–8, 152, 156; and/in microbiome, 151–52; politics of, 6, 14, 96, 101, 105; and vaccines, 21, 37, 78, 90, 91, 92, 96, 100, 103

safety net, 99–100, 176

Samudzi, Zoe, 80

schedules: vaccine, 17, 89, 91, 92n3, 95

science: citizen, 65–66, 105–6; contested, 55, 105; critiques of, 68, 180, 182–83, 184; microbiome, 40, 154, 155; popular, 149, 151, 153; pseudo-, 83, 181; and public reception, 36, 77, 81, 103, 107, 183, 185; and race, 17, 107, 155–56, 185; and rhetorical refusal, 39, 66, 75, 107, 182–85, 186–87; and trust, 91; and vaccine dissent, 65, 77, 79. *See also* biomedical; clinical trials; medicine

schools, 59–60, 127, 161, 164; Waldorf, 24

selective vaccination, 39, 89, 95, 101

side effects. *See* adverse reactions

silence: and/as rhetoric, 27–29, 122–23; and/as rhetorical refusal, 100, 112, 129, 130, 143

Simpson, Audra, 22–24

Smilges, J. Logan, 27, 29, 100

State Medical Review Team (SMRT), 127–29

story: and activism, 63–64; and culture, 61; deep, 97; deficit-based, 126, 129–30, 171; as elicited in healthcare, 172–76; and/as health education, 13; lost, 122, 128, 129–30, 173; personal, 61, 158–65, 174; and power, 34, 74; about Somali Minnesotans, 3–4, 66, 74; and state mediation, 119, 123, 125–29, 141, 173; as surfaced by rhetorical refusal, 75, 108–9, 112, 130, 145; -telling about children, 25, 56, 58, 123, 124–26, 129–30, 170–71, 172, 174–75; -telling about vaccine dissent, 76–77; and/as topos, 172–76, 183; about 2017 Minnesota measles outbreak, 3–5, 74, 82, 84, 87, 101, 108; unfundable/fundable, 126, 127, 130 stock story (term), 34, 66, 87, 128. *See also* counterstory

Sobo, Elisa, 24, 179, 187, 190

social determinants of health, 20–21, 43, 69–70, 96–99, 148–50, 177–79, 180, 182–83

social services: and/for autism, 37, 190, 114–15; and documentation, 116–19, 140–41; and methods, 31–34; and rhetorical refusals, 40, 71; and rules, 119–21, 131–34, 138, 140, 178; and parent interactions, 128–30, 131, 138; and Somali outreach, 110–12, 145–46

Somalis: and autism, 2–5, 2n1, 61, 64–65, 73–74, 98, 115, 159–65, 174; and discrimination, 59, 60–62, 88–100, 94, 96–98; and exclusion, 100–101, 112–13, 122, 168; and health, 90–93, 174, 175–76, 177–79; and precarity, 99–100, 112–13; and racialized surveillance, 59, 70, 80, 124, 126–27, 129, 130, 145, 160, 163; and resettlement, 63, 64, 67, 70, 112–14, 173–74; and school, 96, 99, 101, 122–23, 128–29, 161; services and/for, 110–12, 112–14, 116–19; and support networks, 123, 132, 137, 140, 144, 179–81; and vaccines, 3–5, 81, 88–104, 109, 186

Somalia, 2n2, 58, 93, 98, 113–14

stigma, 52, 56, 57, 58, 129, 186

surveillance, 8–9, 80, 124, 126–27, 129, 130, 160, 163, 173

suspicion, 7, 18, 21–22, 97n5, 190

testimonial injustice (term), 29, 122, 128, 169, 188

Teston, Christa, 28

therapy, 161, 163, 180; behavioral, 37, 47, 50, 115, 132, 136; goat, 170–72; helminthic, 153; medical, 42, 47, 54, 109, 115–16, 130, 166, 180, 185; microbiome, 152–53, 170–72, 181; occupational, 132, 161, 169; speech, 50, 132, 161, 163, 169

topos/topoi, 40, 148, 165–79, 165n3, 181, 182–84, 185, 190

trust: as frame, 7, 12, 16–18, 106; in healthcare relationships, 4, 5, 15, 84, 85, 138, 139, 142, 144, 169, 171–72; and medicine, 66, 98, 99–100, 102; and rhetorical refusal, 148; and the state, 96, 98; and vaccination, 84–86, 89, 91–92, 101

Tuck, Eve, 23, 30

Tuskegee experiments, 96–97

tutoring, 131, 132, 133, 135, 136, 144

undervaccination, 79, 86–87

vaccine hesitancy, 10–11, 16–17, 24, 75, 78, 80, 85–86, 89–99. *See also* antivaccination; fertile ground; vaccines

vaccines: and controversy, 4–5, 74–79, 82–84; and distrust, 63–64, 89–99; and gender, 77–79; in global South, 13, 18, 21–22; public health approaches to, 4–5, 10–11, 17, 74, 84–86, 102; and race, 73, 79–84, 86–87, 94, 96–98; and/for refugees, 25, 84–87, 90, 91–93, 94, 96–98; and rhetorical refusal, 100–108; Somali parent accounts of, 5, 53, 63, 88, 90, 92, 93, 95, 97, 98; and 2017 Minnesota measles outbreak, 2–5, 39, 72–75, 82–86. *See also* antivaccination; measles; measles-mumps-rubella (MMR) vaccine; science

visibility, 27

vitamin D, 48–49, 53, 65

waivers, 111, 138, 162n1

Wakefield study, 76–77, 82, 87

Western disease (term), 41, 42, 58, 66, 128, 157

whiteness, 7, 8, 75, 77, 86–87, 155–56

World Health Organization (WHO), 10–11, 12

writing, 116, 119, 121, 122, 128, 129, 136, 141, 145, 168

Yam, Shui-yin Sharon, 28–29, 176

Yang, K. Wayne, 23, 30

Yergeau, M. Remi, 27–28

Zarowsky, Christina, 68

www.ingramcontent.com/pod-product-compliance
Lightning Source LLC
Chambersburg PA
CBHW020653230426
43665CB00008B/425